To X-Ray, RUH as Bench Book
March 1981

Atlas of
ROENTGENOGRAPHIC MEASUREMENT

*A*tlas of
Roentgenographic

Third

35 EAST WACKER DRIVE • CHICAGO

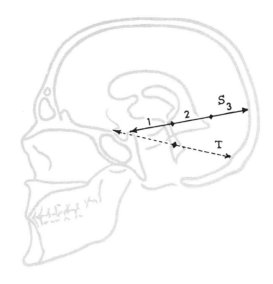

MEASUREMENT

LEE B. LUSTED, M.D.
Professor of Radiology, The University of Chicago

THEODORE E. KEATS, M.D.
Professor and Chairman, Department of Radiology, University of Virginia School of Medicine

Edition

YEAR BOOK MEDICAL PUBLISHERS · INC.

Second Edition, 1967
Third Edition, 1972
Reprinted, August 1973

Library of Congress Catalog Card Number: 70-188576
International Standard Book Number: 0-8151-5654-5

TO

HOWARD L. STEINBACH

Foreword

Since the conception of radiology as a medical science, the growth of this field has been truly remarkable. The early pioneers in the field had little or no knowledge of the normal anatomy or physiology of the living human and, of necessity, relied on morbid anatomy and existing texts. The early radiologic literature was based on empiric observation. These observations, when correlated with what was considered normal in the cadaver, led to erroneous concepts of normal anatomy and physiology.

It soon became apparent that a thorough knowledge of the normal roentgenologic anatomy was necessary before the physician could reliably detect the pathologic state. As a result of intensive studies of normal subjects, a great body of statistics has been accumulated representing the wide range in size and form of normal structures. However, the great number and relative inaccessibility of these observations has precluded their routine use by the busy practitioner of radiology.

This book should be of value to the physician because it provides him, in one volume, the most useful roentgenographic measurements in the medical literature. It should point the way to further studies of a statistical nature in those fields in which there is a lack of information or a conflict of observations.

The selection of the most pertinent information to be included in a book such as this is a difficult task. The authors have done their job well; and it is hoped that they will continue to collect new data, as they become available, for future editions.

HOWARD L. STEINBACH

Preface to Third Edition

The opportunity to prepare a third edition of the *Atlas of Roentgenographic Measurement* has provided the stimulus to review measurements published in the first two editions and to add some new entities. We appreciate the criticisms of reviewers and readers as well as the suggestions about material which should be included.

We wish to emphasize that radiographic measurements are an aid in cases where there is uncertainty about a diagnosis, The measurements listed are the actual measurements taken from the radiograph and a target-film distance is given so that an anatomic measurement can be calculated. For instance, the height of the fourth ventricle of the brain is reported as 14.6 mm. This is the height measured on the film. With a target-film distance of 75 cm. and 11 cm. distance from mid-sagittal plane of skull to film, the magnification factor is 1.17 and the anatomic height of fourth ventricle is 14.6/1.17=12.5 mm. The reader must be cognizant of this element of distortion before applying the data to his own work.

Some measurements which appeared in previous editions have been omitted because better measurements have been published or because the measurements did not seem useful in clinical practice. Other measurements, such as heel pad thickness and chain cystography, remain controversial.

New material has been added to almost all of the chapters, which indicates the continuing interest in the subject of radiographic measurement. However, the useful information to be gained from any radiographic examination must be weighed against the cost in money and radiation exposure to the patient. This benefit-cost relationship is most important to consider in examinations such as pelvimetry and anteversion of the femoral neck because of the high radiation dose inherent in the examination.

Measurements continue to appear on localization of the calcified pineal on the lateral skull roentgenogram. This implies that none of the existing methods is entirely satisfactory. Other new material includes central nervous system measurements, localization of intraocular foreign bodies, cortical bone measurements, information about stereo tube shift and the metric system.

In an attempt to look into the future, we have included probability tables and ultrasonic measurements. This is an experiment and we hope to obtain readers' comments on the usefulness of this type of material.

What future developments in quantitative radiology might be expected to follow data collection from static images? One useful next step would be collection and analysis of radiologic data to construct "public models" as an aid to radiologic diagnosis. Public models usually represent a model, statistical or otherwise, which command general agreement among scientists. The purpose of a public model is to try to reduce disagreement and uncertainty among radiologists about the definition, appearance and probability of radiologic observations. An example is shown in Chapter 6 to illustrate a public model with probability tables to be used in the differentiation of benign versus malignant gastric ulcer. Models of this type could be collected as a part of this *Atlas* or in a separate handbook as an aid to the radiologist and eventually the data could be stored in computer memory.

A word of caution about observer variation and about the application of measurements to a particular patient. The phenomenon of observer variation should be known to most radiologists. Roche *et al.** found that in assessments of skeletal maturity in clinical practice, using the Greulich and Pyle standards for the hand-wrist, the mean absolute differences between repeated assessments by the same observer were about three months. The differences between observers ranged from five weeks to eighteen weeks. Incidentally, Roche and French† found that the median difference in skeletal maturity between the knee and hand was close to zero in normal children and concluded that either of these areas could be assessed as a guide to skeletal maturition in a population study.

Many factors influence the mineral content of bone and thus the radiographic measurement of cortical bone thickness. Virtama and Helelä‡ discuss these factors in their monograph on cortical bone. For instance, they note that the amount of cortical bone in the Finnish population and in individuals of Chinese and Japanese ancestry is less than in Americans of European ancestry. In most cases we have noted the source of material so the radiologist may take population considerations into account.

We are grateful to the many authors who have allowed us to reproduce their original work in the *Atlas* and to the publishers for permission to reproduce the data.

Especially, we thank Shirley A. Nyden, who did the secretarial work on both the second and third editions, and to Charles Wellek for the new illustrations.

LEE B. LUSTED, M.D.
THEODORE E. KEATS, M.D.

---

*Roche, A. F., Davila, G. A., Pasternach, B.A. and Walton, M. J.: Amer J Roentgen 109:299, 1970.

†Roche, A. F. and French, N.Y.: Amer J Roentgen 109:307, 1970.

‡Virtama, P. and Helelä, T.: Acta Radiol, Supp. 293, 1969.

Preface to First Edition

With the discovery of roentgen rays it was possible, for the first time, to make accurate measurements of internal anatomic structures in living subjects. The value of such measurement had been firmly established by the anatomists. It is, therefore, not surprising that the accumulation of roentgen-image measurements was begun and that in a relatively short period of time a great wealth of material was collected.

Because of the large volume of measurement information, it is difficult for the busy practitioner of medicine to find specific data and to recognize that which is valid. Also, it is difficult for him to have at hand the reference material which is necessary in his daily work. These are acute problems for the physician whose practice is not confined to a single location and who does not have a conveniently accessible medical library. This atlas has been compiled to help fill these needs. But, needless to say, the limitation of such an atlas should be recognized by the reader, for it is not possible to present all of the measurements which have been reported. We have included the data that are, in our opinion, most reliable and practical. In some cases the data have a questionable statistical value because of the small sample. In these cases, however, the type of measurement selected was thought to be important and to be the best available.

There are several serious limitations to roentgenographic measurements: first, the roentgenologic image is not sharp; second, the anatomic points for the measurements are not always clearly defined, and they are subject to individual interpretation; and third, in many cases the wide range of normal anatomic variation has not been defined.

The interpretation of a roentgenogram remains an art—an art which depends, in part, upon the Gestalt which the physician has developed from his study of many similar roentgenograms. To this interpretation the objective evidence of the roentgenographic measurement can make an important contribution.

There are several areas of roentgenographic measurement which need further investigation. This is particularly true in pediatrics. Undoubtedly, more measurement data will be forthcoming as the result of the brisk activity in pediatric roentgenology.

We wish to thank Dr. Howard L. Steinbach for directing our attention to the need for such an atlas and for his critical review of the manuscript, and we are indebted to Dr. John F. Holt for his suggestions concerning improvement of this presentation and to the University of Missouri Research Council for financial assistance which helped to make the project possible.

Mr. William E. Loechel, of the National Institute of Health, prepared many of the drawings.

We are grateful to the many authors who have allowed us to reproduce their original work in the *Atlas*, and to their publishers for kind permission to reproduce the data.

Especially, we thank our secretaries—Lecho Otts, Lillian Worden, Josephyne Corsi, and Helena Vatter—for their excellent help in preparing the manuscript.

LEE B. LUSTED
THEODORE E. KEATS

Table of Contents

Geometric Distortion of the Roentgen Image and Its Correction

The roentgen image of an object is larger than the object. This image distortion is caused by the divergence of the roentgen rays, and the amount of distortion is a function of three factors (Fig. 1): the object dimension *(O)*, the target-film distance *(D)*, and the object-film distance *(d)*.

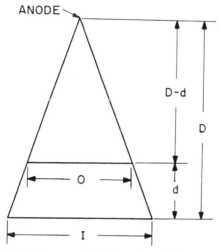

FIG. 1.—(Courtesy of G. H. Brown, Jr. From Am. J. Roentgenol. 78:1063, 1957.)

To find the true object dimension, the image dimension is multiplied by a number less than one (correction factor, *CF*). This correction factor is obtained by means of the following equation, in which

O = Object dimension (cm.)
I = Image dimension on the film (cm.)
D = Target-film distance (cm.)
d = Object-film distance (cm.)

It is important to have all dimensions in the same units. Then, by similar triangles,

$$\frac{O}{I} = \frac{D - d}{D} \qquad \text{and} \qquad O = \frac{(D - d)}{(D)} I$$

Therefore,

$$CF = \frac{D - d}{D}$$

GEOMETRIC DISTORTION OF THE ROENTGEN IMAGE
AND ITS CORRECTION

A number of devices have been constructed which give a fully compensated value of a given object dimension. These devices have usually been made for use in pely-cephalometry.

A nomogram (Fig. 2) and a base chart (Fig. 3) may be used for finding corrected dimensions and for converting a given target-film distance to another target-film distance.

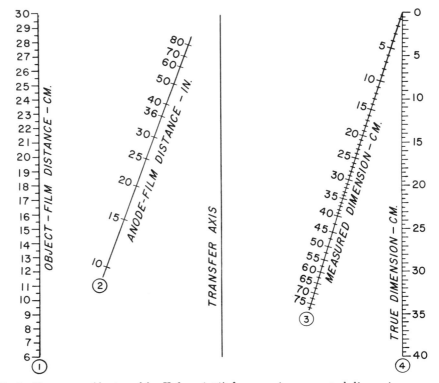

FIG. 2.—Nomogram (designed by Holmquist*) for securing corrected dimensions.

1. Draw a straight line from the object-film distance *(1)* through the anode-film distance *(2)* to the transfer axis.

2. Draw a second line from this point on the transfer axis through the measured dimension *(3)* to the true dimension *(4)*.

*Ball, R. P., and Golden, R.: Am. J. Roentgenol. 49:731 (Fig. 5), 1943.

GEOMETRIC DISTORTION OF THE ROENTGEN IMAGE
AND ITS CORRECTION

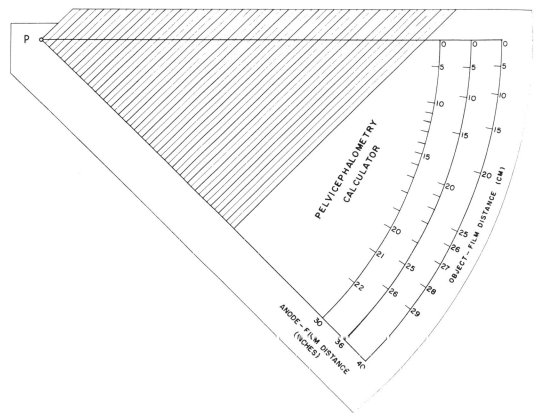

FIG. 3.—Base chart* for constructing a roentgen-image distortion calculator. (Approx. × 1/2.) To use the calculator, a centimeter scale, pivoted at P, is set for the correct object-film distance value, which is located on the appropriate target-film scale. The image dimension is measured on the centimeter scale at the top of the calculator. From the scale point so obtained, the corresponding oblique guide line is followed down to the pivoted centimeter scale. The compensated dimension is read from the centimeter scale at the intersection of the guide line and the pivoted scale.

*Brown, G. H., Jr.: Am. J. Roentgenol. 78:1063 (Fig. 6), 1957.

GEOMETRIC DISTORTION OF THE ROENTGEN IMAGE AND ITS CORRECTION

The following tables can be used for converting centimeters to inches, and inches to centimeters.

CM.	IN.		IN.	CM.
1	0.39		1	2.54
2	0.78		2	5.08
3	1.18		3	7.62
4	1.57		4	10.16
5	1.96		5	12.70
6	2.36		6	15.24
7	2.75		7	17.78
8	3.15		8	20.32
9	3.54		9	22.86
10	3.94		10	25.40
15	5.90		11	27.94
20	7.87		12	30.48
25	9.84		13	33.02
30	11.81		14	35.56
35	13.78		15	38.10
40	15.75		16	40.64
45	17.71		17	43.18
50	19.68		18	45.72
55	21.65		19	48.26
60	23.62		20	50.80
65	25.59		21	53.34
70	27.55		22	55.88
75	29.52		23	58.42
80	31.49		24	60.96
85	33.46		25	63.50
90	35.43		26	66.04
95	37.40		27	68.58
100	39.37		28	71.12
			29	73.66
			30	76.20
			32	81.3
			34	86.4
			36	91.4
			38	96.5
			40	101.6
			48	121.9
			60	152.4
			72	182.9

The amount of shift used to obtain stereo radiographs may be calculated as follows:

$$\frac{\text{Target-film distance}}{\left(\dfrac{\text{Film viewing distance}}{\text{Interpupillary distance}}\right)} = \text{Total tube shift}$$

(Half of shift to each side of midline)

Examples:

1) Target-film distance = 40 inches
   Film viewing distance = 20 inches
   Interpupillary distance = 2.5 inches

   $$\frac{40}{20 \,/\, 2.5} = 5 \text{ inches}$$ (2.5-inch shift to each side of midline)

2) Target-film distance = 72 inches
   Other quantities as above

   $$\frac{72}{20 \,/\, 2.5} = 9 \text{ inches}$$ (4.5-inch shift to each side of midline)

I. THE CENTRAL NERVOUS SYSTEM

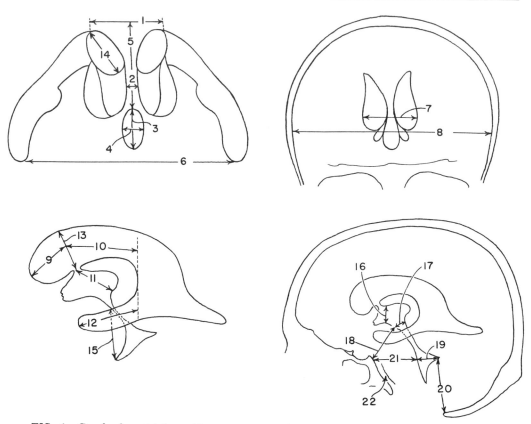

FIG. 4.—Cerebral ventricles. *Top,* anteroposterior projection. *Bottom,* lateral projection. (Redrawn from Orley.)

FIG. 5.—Corpus callosal angle.* *Left,* erect. *Right,* anteroposterior supine. For measurement 23, septum caudate distance, see page 8.

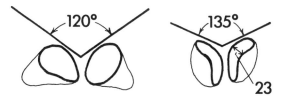

*LeMay, M., and New, P. F. J.: Radiology 96:347, 1970.

MEASUREMENT OF THE CEREBRAL VENTRICLES

DIMENSIONS OF CEREBRAL VENTRICLES—ADULTS*
See Figure 4.

	Lower Limit	Average	Upper Limit
1.		40.0 mm.*	45.0 mm.*
2.		2.5 mm.*	3.0 mm.*
3.		2.0 cm.*	
4.	2.0 mm.‡	7.2 mm. (anterior)‡	10.0 mm.‡
	4.0 mm.‡	8.4 mm. (posterior)‡	10.0 mm.‡
5.		5.0 mm.*	7.0 mm.*
6.		90.0 mm.*	100.0 mm.*
7.		{ratio of 7 to 8 is 0.16-0.29:1}	
8.			
9.		25.0 mm.†	
10.		50.0 mm.†	
11.		26.0 mm.*	
12.		50.0 mm.*	
13.		25.0 mm.*	
14.	16.0 mm.†	18.0 mm.†	20.0 mm.†
15.		40.0 mm.†	
16.	11.0 mm.*	14.2 mm.*	16.0 mm.*
17.	1.0 mm.*	1.5 mm.*	2.0 mm.*
18.	30.0 mm.*	34.4 mm.*	39.0 mm.*
19.	10.0 mm.*	14.6 mm.*	19.0 mm.*
20.	30.0 mm.*	32.6 mm.*	40.0 mm.*
21.	33.3 mm.*	36.1 mm.*	40.0 mm.*
22.	5.0 mm.*	8.2 mm.*	12.0 mm.*

*Davidoff, L. M., and Dyke, C. G.: Am. J. Roentgenol. 44:3, 1940, and *idem, The Normal Pneumoencephalogram* (Philadelphia: Lea & Febiger, 1946).

†Orley, A.: *Neuroradiology* (Springfield, Ill.: Charles C Thomas, Publisher, 1949), pp. 267-268.

‡Borgersen, A.: Acta radiol. (Diagnosis) 4:645, 1966.

Note: Ratios of ventricle-to-skull size are discussed in Berg, K. J., and Lonnum, A.: Acta radiol. (Diagnosis) 4:65, 1966.

DIMENSIONS OF CEREBRAL VENTRICLES–CHILDREN*

See Figure 4.

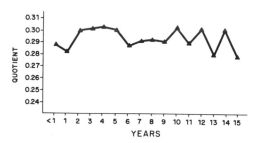

FIG. 6.–Quotient of the anterior horns in the respective age groups. (From Lodin, Fig. 2.)

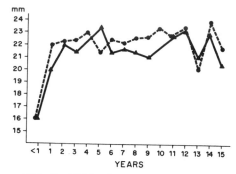

FIG. 7.–Width of anterior horns in mm. Right horn: solid line. Left horn: dotted line. (From Lodin, Fig. 3.)

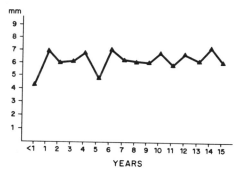

FIG. 8.–Width of 3d ventricle. Measurement 4, Figure 4. (From Lodin, Fig. 4.)

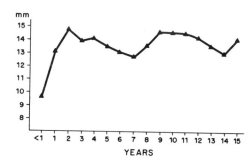

FIG. 9.–Height of 4th ventricle. Measurement 19, Figure 4. (From Lodin, Fig. 6.)

Septum caudate distance: Measurement 23, Figure 5. 10 mm± 0.18 mm. (age 1 year to 15 years). (Lodin)

*Lodin, H.: Acta radiol. (Diagnosis) 7:385, 1968.

MEASUREMENT OF THE CEREBRAL VENTRICLES

1. *Technique*

   a) The anteroposterior projection:
      1. Central ray is vertical and enters a point 3 cm. in front of the root of the nose.
      2. Position: Anteroposterior with patient on his back. Position is correct when the line joining the christa galli and the lambda is perpendicular to a line joining two symmetrical points of the right and left petrous bones.
      3. Target-film distance: 29 inches (Davidoff).
         70 cm. (Orley).
         90 cm. (Lodin).

   b) The lateral projection:
      1. Central ray perpendicular to film centered over midportion of skull.
      2. Position: True lateral.
      3. Target-film distance: 29 inches (Davidoff).
         70 cm. (Orley).
         90 cm. (Lodin).

2. *Measurements*

   See Figure 4.
      1 = Distance between the outermost limits of the bodies at the lateral angles.
      2 = Width of the shadow of the septum pellucidum.
      3 = Vertical diameter of the 3d ventricle.
      4 = Width of the shadow of the 3d ventricle.
      5 = Distance between the tips of the lateral ventricles and the dorsal end of the shadow of the septum pellucidum.
      6 = Distance between the two temporal horns.
      7 = Transverse diameter of the anterior horns.
      8 = Transverse diameter of the skull.
      9 = Average length of the anterior horn of the lateral ventricle.
      10 = Length of the body of the lateral ventricle.
      11 = Diagonal distance between the foramen of Monro and the rostral end of the aqueduct of Sylvius.
      12 = Length of the temporal horn of the lateral ventricle.
      13 = Distance from the foramen of Monro to the roof of the lateral ventricle.
      14 = Diagonal width of the body of the lateral ventricle.
      15 = Caudal end of the 4th ventricle to the cephalic end of the aqueduct of Sylvius.
      16 = Prepineal ventrodorsal diameter of the 3d ventricle.
      17 = Height of the aqueduct of Sylvius.
      18 = Distance from the aqueduct of Sylvius to the dorsum sellae.
      19 = Maximum height of the 4th ventricle.
      20 = Distance between the superior recess of the 4th ventricle and the floor of the skull.
      21 = Distance from the dorsum sellae to the floor of the 4th ventricle at the level of the superior recess.
      22 = Distance from the dorsum sellae to the anterior margin of the pons varolii.

3. *Source of Material*

   The dimensions of Davidoff and Dyke were based on 150 encephalograms in which the size of the ventricles appeared to correspond to the accepted size for the normal in standard books on anatomy.

   Orley states that the number of encephalograms measured was "fairly substantial."

POSITION OF THE AQUEDUCT AND FOURTH VENTRICLE*

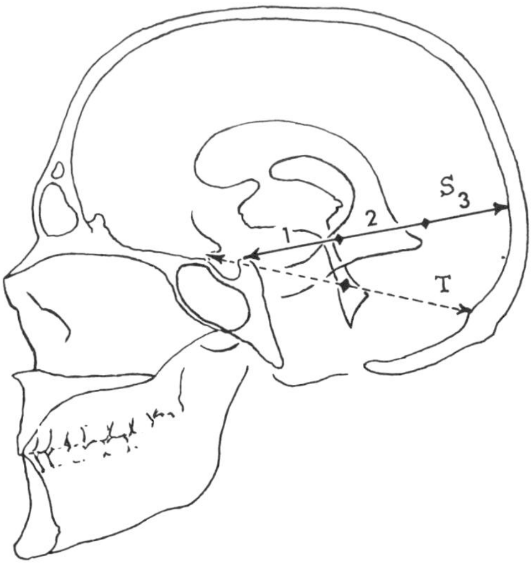

FIG. 10.—Swedish line[†] and Twining line.[‡] The Swedish line *(S)* (modified from Sahlstedt) is drawn from the tip of the dorsum sellae through the lower part of the aqueduct to the skull vault. The Twining line *(T)* is drawn from the tuberculum sellae to the internal occipital protuberance.

1. *Technique*

a) Central ray: Perpendicular to the film centered 1 inch anterior and 1 inch superior to external auditory meatus.

b) Position: True lateral of skull (3d ventricle and 4th ventricle—views of the pneumoencephalogram or ventriculogram).

c) Target-film distance: 75 cm. used by Sutton, but distance not critical for this study.

2. *Measurements*

a) **Position of the aqueduct:**

Divide line S (Fig. 10) into three parts. The aqueduct will lie at about the junction of the first and middle thirds.

b) **Position of the 4th ventricle:**

Bisect line T. The midpoint of line T should lie within the 4th ventricle.

Displacement of the aqueduct or 4th ventricle in the lateral projection is helpful in detecting subtentorial lesions.

3. *Source of Material*

Sutton's encephalograms of 100 normal cases were used as a basis. Sutton found no case where the aqueduct was above the junction of the first and middle thirds of the Swedish line. The midpoint of Twining's line lay in the 4th ventricle or posterior to the floor of the 4th ventricle in all 100 cases.

Note:

A ratio $= \dfrac{\text{Distance of nasion-inion}}{\text{Distance of inion-foramen magnum}}$ has been used by Schechter and
$\qquad\qquad\qquad\qquad$ (posterior lip)

Zingesser (Radiology 88:905, 1967) in cases of aqueductal stenosis. Normal value of the ratio is 3; for aqueductal stenosis cases the ratio range is 4 to 7.5 (Wolpert, S. M.: Radiology 92:1511, 1969.)

---

*Sutton, D.: Brit. J. Radiol. 23:208, 1950.

[†]Sahlstedt, H.: Acta radiol., supp. 24, 1935.

[‡]Twining, E. W.: Brit. J. Radiol. 12:569, 1939.

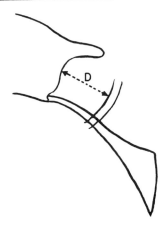

FIG. 11—(Redrawn from Klaus.)

1. *Technique*

    a) Central ray: Perpendicular to film. Center is 1 inch anterior to and 1 inch superior to external auditory meatus.

    b) Position: True lateral pneumoencephalogram.

    c) Target-film distance: 75 cm.

2. *Measurements*

    See Figure 11. Distance D is the shortest distance between the posterior margin of the 3d ventricle and the ambient cistern. Normal range, 7-14 mm.

3. *Source of Material*

    Two hundred normal adult pneumoencephalograms were used as a basis.

*Klaus, E.: Acta radiol. 50:12, 1958.

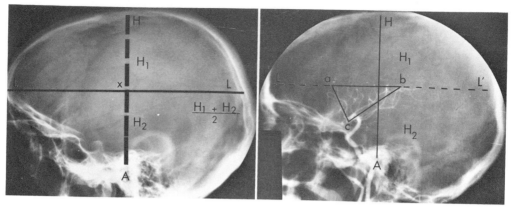

FIG. 12.   FIG. 13.

Lines of reference to determine displacement of the superior insular line on the vertical plane.

Lines of reference to determine displacement of the triangle on the sagittal plane. (Figs. 12-15 are from Gonzalez *et al.*, Figs. 1-4.)

FIG. 14.   FIG. 15.

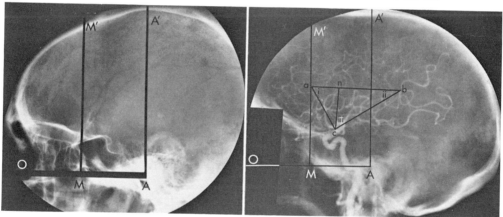

1. Technique

   a) Central ray: To a point 1 inch anterior and 1 inch superior to external auditory meatus.

   b) Position: True lateral carotid arteriogram.

   c) Target-film distance: 44 inches.

2. Measurements

   a) Construction of the sylvian triangle.
      See Figures 13 and 15.

   ab = Superior insular line or sylvian line. Line joining the highest points of the first loops of the insular arteries, excepting the first, the fronto-orbital.

   bc = Lower border of triangle. A line along the segment of the middle cerebral artery lying within the sylvian fissure. This line joins the origin of the first superior branch of the artery to the highest point of the curve of the middle cerebral trunk.

   ac = Anterior border of triangle. A line joining the origin of the first superior branch (the inferior point, c) to the most antero-superior vascular loop.

---

*Fernandez-Servats, A. A.; Vlahovitch, B.; and Parker, S. A.: J. Neurol. Neurosurg. & Psychiat. 31:379, 1968.

†Gonzalez, C.; Kricheff, I. I.; Lin, J. P.; and Lorber, S.: Radiology 94:535, 1970.

b) Construction of reference lines.

See Figures 12 and 13.

AH = Hemisphere height. Line from superior border of the external auditory meatus to inner table of the skull. Line is drawn perpendicular to sylvian line, *ab*. AH is divided by the sylvian line into two portions, H_1 and H_2 which are used to determine variations of the sylvian triangle in the vertical plane.

See Figures 14 and 15.

OA = Anthropometric base line (Frankfurt plane). Line from orbital floor (O) to superior border of external auditory meatus (A).

AA^1 = Intraauricular line. Line perpendicular to line OA at the level of the external auditory meatus.

MM^1 = Line perpendicular to line OA halfway between points O and A.

c) Extremities of the sylvian triangle.

See Figure 15.

	Gonzalez et al.	*Vlahovitch*
Point *a*:	1.31 mm. (S.D. ± 1.72 mm.) posterior to MM^1	0.57 mm. (S.D. ± 2.27 mm.) posterior to MM^1
Point *b*:	5 to 25 mm. posterior to AA^1	10 to 25 mm. posterior to AA^1
Point *c*:	Within ± 4.5 mm. in any direction from a point at the junction of lower one fourth of AA^1 and posterior one third of OA.	

d) Angles of the sylvian triangle.

See Figure 15

	Vlahovitch	*Gonzalez* et al.
Anterosuperior angle (i) =	65° (P-95_ ± 11°)	61° (P-95_ ± 12°)
Posterior angle (ii) =	30° (P-95_ ± 7.8°)	35° (P-95_ ± 21°)
Inferior angle (iii) =	85° (P-95_ ± 10°)	79° (P-95_ ± 15°)

(From Gonzalez *et al.*, Table 1.)

e) Height of the sylvian triangle.

See Figure 15. Height *cn* is one-fourth the hemisphere height, AH.

f) Superior border of the sylvian triangle.

See Figures 12 and 13.

The superior insular line is at one-half the hemisphere height, *AH*. Standard deviation is 2.5 mm. In 95% of cases the superior insular line will lie within 5 mm. of point *x*.

TABULATION OF SUPERIOR INSULAR LINE RELATIVE TO HEMISPHERE HEIGHT WITH CALCULATION OF STANDARD DEVIATIONS

Height of Hemisphere	Position of Superior Insular Line (S.D. = 1σ)	Position of Superior Insular Line (S.D. = 2σ)
11	5.60 ± 0.40	5.60 ± 0.80
12	5.90 ± 0.21	5.90 ± 0.42
12.2	6.10 ± 0.25	6.10 ± 0.52
12.3	6.00 ± 0.11	6.00 ± 0.22
12.5	6.27 ± 0.11	6.27 ± 0.22
12.8	6.30 ± 0.14	6.30 ± 0.28
13.0	6.57 ± 0.28	6.57 ± 0.56
13.4	6.36 ± 0.35	6.36 ± 0.70
13.5	6.77 ± 0.26	6.77 ± 0.52
14.0	6.96 ± 0.23	6.96 ± 0.46
14.5	7.12 ± 0.25	7.12 ± 0.50
Av. SD	±0.23	± 0.47

(From Gonzalez *et al.*, Table 2.)

Particular attention should be given to displacement of the superior insular line. Concavity in any border of the triangle or deformation of the angles of the triangle is found with space-occupying lesions.

Rotation of the skull changes all the normal relationships and makes the measurements worthless.

3. *Source of Material*

Fernandez-Serrats, Vlahovitch and Parker studied 100 normal angiograms. Gonzalez *et al.* studied 100 normal angiograms.

SIZE OF THE INTERNAL CAROTID, MIDDLE CEREBRAL
AND ANTERIOR CEREBRAL ARTERIES*

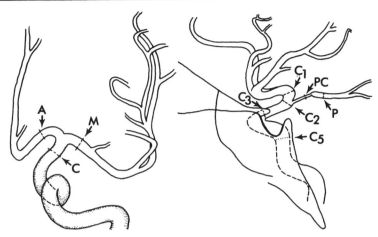

FIG. 16.—(Redrawn from Gabrielsen and Greitz, Figs. 1 and 2.)

1. Technique

   a) Central ray: Anteroposterior—Directed to superior forehead with the beam angulated
      20° cranially.
      Lateral—Perpendicular to the film centered 1 inch anterior and 1 inch
      superior to the external auditory meatus.
   b) Position: Anteroposterior and lateral.
   c) Target-film distance: 85 cm. using a 10 by-12-inch Elema-Schönander film changer.

2. Measurements

See Figure 16.

Anteroposterior view:

C = Diameter of internal carotid artery 5 mm. proximal to its bifurcation into the
   anterior and middle cerebral arteries.

A = Diameter of the anterior cerebral artery 5 mm. distal to origin.

M = Diameter of the middle cerebral artery 5 mm. distal to origin.

Lateral view:

C_1 = Diameter of the internal carotid artery 5 mm. distal to its junction with the
   posterior communicating artery.

C_2 = Diameter of the internal carotid artery just proximal to the junction with the
   posterior communicating artery.

C_3 = Diameter of the internal carotid artery at the level of the tuberculum sellae.

C_5 = Diameter of the internal carotid artery just proximal to its bend at the posterior
   aspect of the cavernous sinus.

C_6 = Diameter of the internal carotid artery at the level of the atlas.

PC = Diameter of the posterior communication artery 5 mm. distal to its junction with
   the internal carotid artery.

P = Diameter of the posterior cerebral artery 5 mm. distal to its junction with the
   posterior communicating artery.

*Gabrielsen, T. O., and Greitz, T.: Acta radiol. (Diagnosis) 10:1, 1970.

SIZE OF THE INTERNAL CAROTID, MIDDLE CEREBRAL AND ANTERIOR CEREBRAL ARTERIES

MEAN VALUES FOR VARIOUS DIAMETERS OF NORMAL CEREBRAL ARTERIES

Measurement	Mean Diameter	S.D.
M	3.82 mm.	0.43 mm.
A	3.02 mm.	0.50 mm.
C	4.57 mm.	0.46 mm.
C_1	3.78 mm.	0.43 mm.
C_2	4.08 mm.	0.47 mm.
C_3	5.12 mm.	0.63 mm.
C_5	5.80 mm.	0.76 mm.
C_6	5.90 mm.	0.73 mm.
Siphon length	15.1 mm.	2.45 mm.

Based on 156 normal carotid angiographies.
No correction for sex and skull size.

(From Gabrielsen and Greitz, Table 1.)

INFLUENCE OF SEX AND EXTERNAL BIPARIETAL DIAMETER (W IN CM.) ON SIZE OF INTERNAL CAROTID AND MIDDLE CEREBRAL ARTERIES (IN MM.)

Measurement	Male	Female
M	$1.97 + 0.118\,W$	$1.78 + 0.118\,W$
C	$2.99 + 0.100\,W$	$2.81 + 0.100\,W$
C_5	$4.56 + 0.112\,W$	$3.91 + 0.112\,W$
$M + C + C_5$	$9.52 + 0.330\,W$	$8.50 + 0.330\,W$

(From Gabrielsen and Greitz, Table 2.)

3. *Source of Material*

One hundred fifty-six angiograms from 72 males and 84 females, ranging in age from 13 to 69 years. Mean age was 33 years. Great care was taken to select normal cases. Excluded from the study were cases with even minimal atherosclerosis, cerebral spasm.

A series of test films for calibrating films may on request be obtained from Prof. T. Greitz, Karolinska sjukhuset 104-01 Stockholm 60, Sweden.

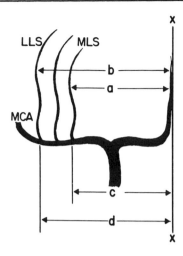

FIG. 17.—(Redrawn from Anderson.)

1. *Technique*

   a) Central ray: Vertical and enters a point 3 cm. in front of the root of the nose.

   b) Position: Anteroposterior.

   c) Target-film distance: 75 cm.

2. *Measurements*

   See Figure 17.

   X = Midplane of skull.

   MLS = Most medial lenticulostriate artery.

   LLS = Most lateral lenticulostriate artery.

   MCA = Middle cerebral artery.

DISTANCES	AVERAGE NORMAL VALUES
$a =$	26 mm.
$b =$	38 mm.
$c =$	17 mm.
$d =$	30 mm.

3. *Source of Material*

   Studies were made of an unselected series of 300 consecutive adult carotid angiographies.

---

*Anderson, P. E.: Acta radiol. 50:84, 1958.

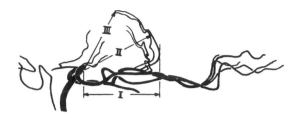

FIG. 18.—(From Lofgen, p. 111.)

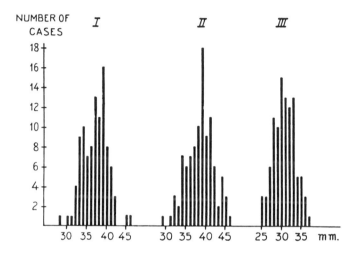

FIG. 19.—(From Lofgren, p. 113.)

1. *Technique*

   a) Central ray: To a point 1 inch anterior to and 1 inch superior to external auditory meatus.

   b) Position: Lateral.

   c) Target-film distance: 75 cm.

2. *Measurements*

   See Figures 18 and 19.

   Distance measured from bifurcation between the basilar artery and the posterior cerebellar artery:
   I. To the tangent to the posterior part of the choroid artery as measured along a line parallel to the longitudinal direction of the posterior cerebral artery.
   II. To (the greatest distance) the posterior choroid artery.
   III. To the anterior upper part of the posterior choroid artery.

3. *Source of Material*

   One hundred normal adult vertebral arteriograms were studied.

---

*Lofgren, F. O.: Acta radiol. 50:108, 1958.

MEASUREMENT OF THE VENOUS ANGLE OF THE BRAIN*

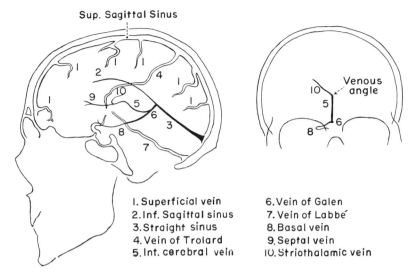

FIG. 20.—Deep venous circulation of brain.

1. Superficial vein   6. Vein of Galen
2. Inf. Sagittal sinus   7. Vein of Labbé
3. Straight sinus   8. Basal vein
4. Vein of Trolard   9. Septal vein
5. Int. cerebral vein   10. Striothalamic vein

FIG. 21.—(Redrawn from Probst, Fig. 5.)

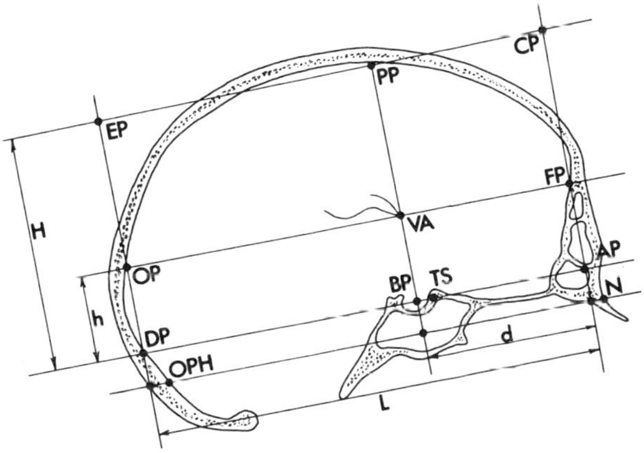

1. *Technique*

   a) Central ray: To a point 1 inch anterior and 1 inch superior to the external
   auditory meatus.

   b) Position: True lateral.

   c) Target-film distance: 100 cm.

2. *Measurements*

   See Figure 21.

   a) Construction of reference lines:

   Line *N-OPH* = A line from nasion to opisthion.

   Line *AP-TS* = Base line drawn parallel to line *N-OPH* through the tuberculum
   sellae *(TS)*.

   Line *FP-VA* = Venous angle horizontal line is drawn parallel to line *N-OPH*
   through the venous angle *(VA)*. *VA* is the point at which the
   striothalamic vein joins the internal cerebral vein. The anterior

*Probst, F. P.: Acta radiol. (Diagnosis) 10:271, 1970.

convexity point is usually directed anteriorly, but it may point anteroinferiorly. If the angle takes the form of a large arc, one should choose the anteroinferior convexity point of the arc for the orientation study.

Line CP-PP = Parietal line drawn parallel to line N-OPH through a point on the inner table of the parietal bone (PP).

Line AP-CP = Frontal line drawn perpendicular to line N-OPH through a point on the inner table of the frontal bone (FP).

Line BP-PP = Venous angle vertical line drawn perpendicular to line N-OPH through point VA.

Line DP-EP = Occipital line drawn perpendicular to line N-OPH through a point on the inner table at the occipital bone (OP).

b) Measure the following lengths in millimeters:

Frontal distance (d) = FP-VA.
Total length (L) = FP-OP.
Basal distance (h) = BP-VA.
Total height (H) = BP-PP.

Plot the distances on the two charts in Figure 22.

The two charts are integrated in Figure 23.

The regression line in each chart in Figure 22 is identical with the y and x axes, respectively, in Figure 23.

The range of variation is indicated by the ellipses in Figure 23: 99% of normals $(P = 0.01)$ will fall inside the larger ellipse and 95% of normals $(P = 0.05)$ will fall inside the smaller ellipse.

FIG. 22.—(Redrawn from Probst, Fig. 6.)

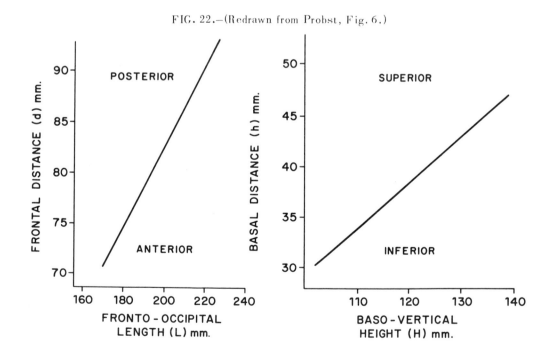

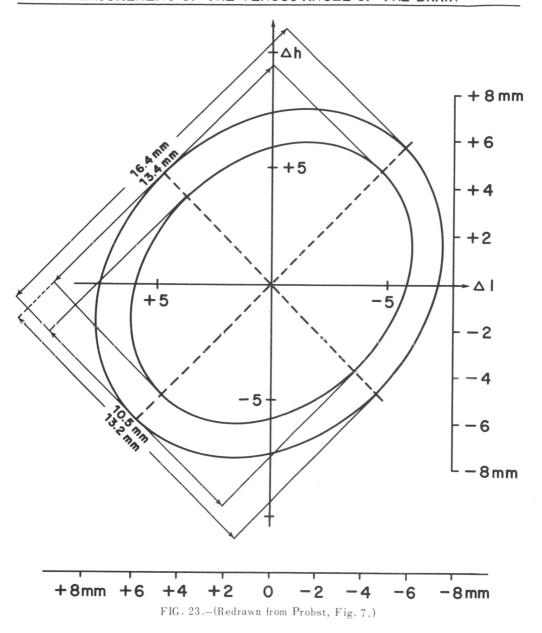

FIG. 23.—(Redrawn from Probst, Fig. 7.)

3. Source of Material

Two hundred sixteen carotid angiograms from adults judged to be normal.

CIRCULATION TIME IN VESSELS OF THE BRAIN*

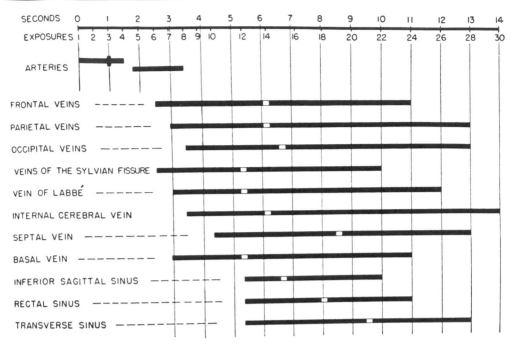

FIG. 24.—Sequence of contrast filling of different veins in the normal case. The lines are broken at the point of maximum filling, i.e., the transition between filling and emptying phases. This point determined for parietal veins, roughly coincides with the average for cerebral veins. (From Greitz, diag. 1.)

1. *Technique*
   a) Central ray: To a point 1 inch anterior and 1 inch superior to external auditory meatus.
   b) Position: Lateral.
   c) Target-film distance: Immaterial.

2. *Measurements*

   See Figure 24.

   The head of the column of contrast medium is taken as the point of reference for the measurement of the arterial filling phase, the arterial emptying phase, the venous filling phase, and the venous emptying phase. It is not possible to determine with accuracy the termination of the emptying phase, since the contrast filling seems to decrease asymptotically.

   For this study, Greitz used a cut-film changer with a program technique: 2 films/sec. for the first 5 seconds and then 1 film/sec. for 10 seconds.

3. *Source of Material*

   Cerebral arteriograms from 120 cases were studied.

*Greitz, T.; Acta radiol. 46:285, 1956.

II. THE NECK

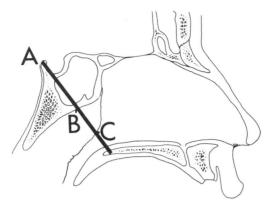

FIG. 25.—(Redrawn from Capitanio and Kirkpatrick, Fig. 2, *B.*)

1. Technique

a) Central ray: To nasopharynx at level of the posterior angle of the mandible.
b) Position: True lateral of the nasopharynx.
c) Target-film distance: 72 inches.

2. Measurements

See Figure 25.

AC = Line from the posterior clinoids perpendicular to the base of the sphenoid bone to the soft-tissue margin outlined by air in the nasopharynx. Radiographs should be exposed in the inspiration phase of respiration and with the mouth open.

BC = Thickness of nasopharyngeal soft tissue.

Age	Infants	Proportion of Infants Showing Thickness of Soft Tissue		
		0.0 mm.	*5 mm. or less*	*5 mm. or more*
1 day— 1 month	36	36/36	0/36	0/36
1— 3 months	76	36/76	39/76	1/76
3— 6 months	47	7/47	25/47	15/47
6—12 months	56	0/56	16/56	40/56
12—24 months	42	0/42	3/42	39/42

3. Source of Material

Two hundred fifty-seven children from age 1 day to 24 months. No child had an immunologic deficiency.

*Capitanio, M. A., and Kirkpatrick, J. A.: Radiology 96:389, 1970.

MEASUREMENT OF THE SOFT TISSUES OF THE NECK*

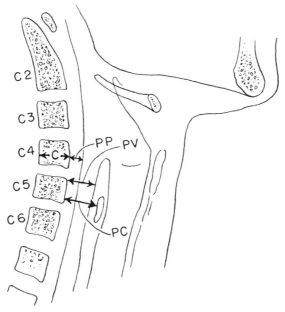

FIG. 26.—(Redrawn from Hay.)

1. *Technique*

 a) Central ray: On coronal plane at the level of the thyroid cartilage.
 b) Position: True lateral.
 c) Target-film distance: 48 inches.

2. *Measurements*

 See Figure 26.

  PV = Postventricular soft tissue.
  PP = Postpharyngeal soft tissue.
  PC = Postcricoid soft tissue.
  C = Anteroposterior dimension of C4 vertebral body at its middle.

---

*Hay, P. D.: "The Neck," in *Annals of Roentgenology*, Vol. 9 (New York: Paul B. Hoeber, Inc., 1939).

MEASUREMENT OF THE SOFT TISSUES OF THE NECK

UPPER NORMAL LIMITS OF SOFT-TISSUE SPACES OF NECK

AGE	POSTPHARYNGEAL SOFT TISSUE			POSTLARYNGEAL SOFT TISSUE	
	POSTVENTRICULAR				
0-1	1.5C4			2.0C4	
1-2	0.5C4			1.5C4	
2-3	0.5C4			1.2C4	
3-6	0.4C4			1.2C4	
6-14	0.3C4			1.2C4	
	POSTCRICOID				
	Male	Female		Male	Female
Adult	0.3C4	0.3C4		0.7C4	0.6C4

All measurements are given as multiples of the AP width of C4 body.

The adult anteroposterior diameter of the trachea at the point of greatest constriction equals 1.2C4.

The retrotracheal space equals 0.6C4.

3. *Source of Material*

Fifty normal adults and 25 normal infants were studied. The 50 normal adults were all examined laryngoscopically. The findings in most of the patients were entirely negative by laryngoscopy, but a few patients showed a slight hyperemia of the mucosa.

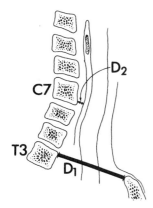

FIG. 27.—(Redrawn from Kendall, Ashcroft and
Whiteside, Fig. 8.)

1. *Technique*

   a) Central ray: Perpendicular to plane of the film directed to the level of the 7th
   cervical and 1st thoracic vertebrae.

   b) Position· True lateral.

   c) Target-film distance: 72 inches

2. *Measurements*

   See Figure 27.

   D_1 = Minimum distance between posterior cortex of manubrium and spine.
   D_2 = Minimum distance between trachea and spine.

Sagittal Inlet (D_1)	*Distance from Spine to Trachea (D_2)*
Average = 6.2 cm.	Average = 1.3 cm.
Range = 5.0 to 8.7 cm.	Range = 0.5 to 2.5 cm.

3. *Source of Material*

   67 patients who had routine barium swallows.

   Note:

   A narrow thoracic inlet may cause compression of the esophagus by the
   trachea. This compression is seen as a smooth, crescent-shaped defect on the
   barium-filled esophagus at the C7 to T3 level. The defect usually is on the
   right side of the esophagus in the posteroanterior projection.

---

*Kendall, B. E.; Ashcroft, K.; and Whiteside, C. G.: Brit. J. Radiol 35:769, 1962.

III. THE SKELETAL SYSTEM

A. The Skull

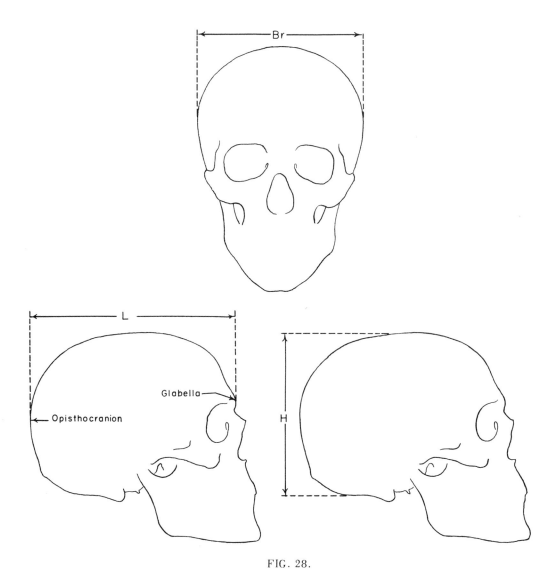

FIG. 28.

MEASUREMENT OF THE NORMAL SKULL*

1. *Technique*

   a) Central ray: Posteroanterior—To glabella.

   Lateral—To a point 1 inch anterior and 1 inch superior to external auditory meatus.

   b) Positions: Posteroanterior.

   Lateral.

   c) Target-table distance: 91.4 cm. (36 inches).

   Table-film distance: 5.6 cm. (Enlargement factor of 16%.)

   Target-film distance: 97.0 cm. (38 inches).

2. *Measurements*

   See Figure 28.

   Br = Greatest transverse diameter of skull in posteroanterior position.

   L = Greatest length of skull = Distance from the glabella to the opisthocranion.

   H = Height of skull = Total height from the basion to the vertex.

   Note:

   a) In roentgenograms the breadth averages from 4 to 8 mm. less on the anteroposterior view than on the posteroanterior view.

   b) Haas feels that it is best to measure breadth at the upper margin of the squamous suture, or slightly above it at the level of the stephanion, when the skull is wider there.

   The modulus $M = \dfrac{L+H+Br}{3}$ is a better indicator of skull size than a single diameter. The computed modulus values conform to anthropologic data.

   The cephalic index, $CI = (Br_L \times 100)$, is characteristic of skull shape.

   Mesocephalic skull, CI = 75-84.

   Brachycephalic skull, CI = 84 or greater.

   Dolichocephalic skull, CI = 75 or less.

   Skull size and measurements have diagnostic value. Deformity itself does not necessarily mean clinical pathology, but deviations in size call for detailed clinical and roentgenologic studies.

   In the tables which follow on pages 32-34.

   $$\text{Modulus } (M) = \frac{L + H + Br}{3} \qquad \text{Cephalic index } (CI) = \frac{Br}{L} \times 100$$

   $V_{min} - V_{max}$ = Variation range from minimum to maximum. Values outside this range are definitely abnormal.

   Adults· $M \pm \sigma$ = Range of variation for mesocephalic skull; σ (standard deviation) not computed for children.

   Values of M outside of $M \pm 2\sigma$ indicate hyperdolichocephaly, and in adults suggest previous pathology in childhood.

   N = number of individuals.

3. *Source of Material*

   Studies were made of 1,300 racially mixed patients of various age groups and both sexes.

---

*Haas, L. L. : Am. J. Roentgenol. 67:197, 1952.

MEASUREMENT OF THE NORMAL SKULL

BREADTH (CM.) OF SKULL ON ROENTGENOGRAMS (DISTORTION: 16 PER CENT)

Age	Male			Female			Total		
	n	$V_{min}-V_{max}$	M	n	$V_{min}-V_{max}$	M	n	$V_{min}-V_{max}$	M
−4 wk.	2	11.1−11.6	11.3	3	10.0−12.0	10.8	5	10.0−12.0	11.0
2−6 mo.	8	11.0−14.1	12.2	7	10.1−12.8	11.6	15	10.1−12.8	11.9
7−12 mo.	14	12.7−15.6	13.9	12	12.0−15.0	13.2	26	12.0−15.6	13.6
13−18 mo.	12	12.8−15.8	14.1	17	12.4−15.6	13.9	29	12.4−15.8	14.0
19−30 mo.	22	14.0−16.7	15.1	9	13.2−16.0	14.4	31	13.2−16.7	14.9
3−5 yr.	38	14.1−17.0	15.3	30	13.1−16.4	14.9	68	13.1−17.0	15.1
6−8 yr.	32	14.1−17.2	15.9	27	13.6−16.6	15.3	59	13.6−17.2	15.6
9−11 yr.	29	14.9−17.6	16.0	23	14.3−17.2	15.5	52	14.3−17.6	15.8
12−14 yr.	29	15.2−17.3	16.2	23	14.7−17.0	15.7	52	14.7−17.3	16.0
15−17 yr.	32	15.0−17.8	16.5	18	14.7−17.1	15.7	50	14.7−17.8	16.2
18−20 yr.	31	14.7−18.9	16.5	24	15.5−17.2	16.1	55	14.7−18.9	16.3
21−	369	14.9−19.0	16.8	356	14.2−17.9	16.2	725	14.2−19.0	16.5
	$\sigma = -0.79 + 0.65$			$\sigma = -0.43 + 0.65$					
	$M \pm \sigma = 16.0-17.4 = 70.9\%$			$M \pm \sigma = 15.4-16.8 = 65.7\%$					
	$M \pm 2\sigma = 15.2-18.1 = 95.4\%$			$M \pm 2\sigma = 14.7-17.4 = 96.3\%$					
TOTAL	618			549			1167		

From Haas, L. L.: Am. J. Roentgenol. 67:197 (Table IV), 1952.

LENGTH DIAMETER (CM.) OF RACIALLY MIXED SKULLS ON ROENTGENOGRAMS (DISTORTION: 16 PER CENT) OF VARIOUS AGE GROUPS OF BOTH SEXES

Age	Male			Female			Total		
	n	$V_{min}-V_{max}$	M	n	$V_{min}-V_{max}$	M	n	$V_{min}-V_{max}$	M
−4 wk.	2	13.7−14.2	13.9	3	12.6−14.0	13.2	5	12.6−14.2	13.5
2−6 mo.	8	13.5−16.2	14.7	7	13.4−14.8	14.3	15	13.4−15.0	14.5
7−12 mo.	14	14.0−17.8	16.4	12	14.5−16.9	15.8	26	14.0−17.6	16.1
13−18 mo.	12	15.8−18.2	17.1	17	15.8−18.1	17.1	29	15.8−18.2	17.1
19−30 mo.	22	16.1−19.8	18.1	12	15.7−19.5	17.7	34	15.7−19.8	17.9
3−5 yr.	40	16.4−20.4	18.9	30	16.2−20.4	18.8	70	16.2−20.4	18.8
6−8 yr.	33	17.1−20.8	19.4	29	16.0−20.7	19.0	62	16.0−20.8	19.2
9−11 yr.	34	17.9−21.1	19.6	26	16.6−21.3	19.3	60	16.6−21.3	19.5
12−14 yr.	32	18.3−21.8	20.3	26	17.9−21.0	19.7	58	17.9−21.8	20.0
15−17 yr.	34	19.0−22.2	20.6	20	18.7−21.8	20.1	54	18.7−22.2	20.4
18−20 yr.	33	19.6−22.6	20.8	29	19.2−21.0	20.1	62	19.2−22.6	20.5
21−	395	18.9−23.2	21.2	363	18.0−22.3	20.1	758	18.0−23.2	20.7
	$\sigma = -8.0 + 7.9$			$\sigma = -7.5 + 7.4$					
	$M \pm \sigma = 20.4-22.0 = 69.8\%$			$M \pm \sigma = 19.4-20.9 = 74.5\%$					
	$M \pm 2\sigma = 19.6-22.8 = 96.7\%$			$M \pm 2\sigma = 18.7-21.6 = 95.5\%$					
TOTAL	659			574			1233		

From Haas, L. L.: Am. J. Roentgenol. 67:197 (Table II), 1952.

MEASUREMENT OF THE NORMAL SKULL

HEIGHT (CM.) OF SKULL ON ROENTGENOGRAMS (ROENTGENOLOGICAL ENLARGEMENT: 16 PER CENT)

Age	Male			Female			Total		
	n	$V_{min}-V_{max}$	M	n	$V_{min}-V_{max}$	M	n	$V_{min}-V_{max}$	M
−4 wk.	2	10.2−11.2	10.7	3	9.8−13.0	11.1	5	9.8−13.0	11.0
2−6 mo.	8	10.5−13.7	11.7	7	10.8−13.5	11.8	15	10.5−13.7	11.7
7−12 mo.	10	12.1−14.3	13.3	12	11.4−13.6	12.4	22	11.4−14.3	12.8
13−18 mo.	9	12.6−15.0	14.0	17	12.1−15.5	13.6	26	12.1−15.5	13.8
19−30 mo.	22	13.6−15.7	14.7	9	13.2−15.3	14.2	31	13.2−15.7	14.5
3−5 yr.	40	13.5−16.3	14.9	26	13.5−16.0	14.6	66	13.5−16.3	14.7
6−8 yr.	33	14.2−16.7	15.2	27	13.2−16.3	14.8	60	13.2−16.7	15.1
9−11 yr.	34	14.0−17.0	15.3	25	13.8−15.8	14.8	59	13.8−17.0	15.1
12−14 yr.	32	14.4−17.0	15.6	24	13.8−16.3	15.1	56	13.8−17.0	15.4
15−17 yr.	32	14.5−17.1	15.7	19	13.8−15.7	15.0	51	13.8−17.1	15.4
18−20 yr.	29	14.0−17.4	15.6	26	13.0−16.3	15.1	55	13.0−17.4	15.4
21−	379	13.4−17.7	15.6	353	13.4−17.1	15.1	732	13.4−17.7	15.3
	$\sigma = -0.72 + 0.68$			$\sigma = -0.64 + 0.64$					
	$M \pm \sigma = 14.9-16.3 = 75.7\%$			$M \pm \sigma = 14.5-15.8 = 70.0\%$					
	$M \pm 2\sigma = 14.1-16.9 = 95.0\%$			$M \pm 2\sigma = 13.8-16.4 = 95.3\%$					
TOTAL	630			540			1178		

From Haas, L. L.: Am. J. Roentgenol. 67:197 (Table III), 1952.

MODULUS (CM.) OF SKULL ON ROENTGENOGRAMS

Age	Male			Female			Total		
	n	$V_{min}-V_{max}$	M	n	$V_{min}-V_{max}$	M	n	$V_{min}-V_{max}$	M
−4 wk.	2	11.6−12.3	12.0	3	10.8−12.8	11.6	5	10.8−12.3	11.8
2−6 mo.	8	11.9−14.6	12.9	7	12.1−14.1	12.7	15	11.9−14.6	12.8
7−12 mo.	11	13.0−15.3	14.9	12	12.9−15.0	13.8	23	12.9−15.3	14.2
13−18 mo.	9	14.3−16.1	15.3	17	13.5−16.0	14.8	26	13.5−16.1	15.0
19−30 mo.	23	14.5−16.8	15.9	12	13.6−16.6	15.1	35	13.6−16.8	15.7
3−5 yr.	33	14.8−17.4	16.3	26	14.2−17.4	16.0	59	14.2−17.4	16.2
6−8 yr.	29	15.5−17.7	16.8	27	14.3−17.5	16.3	56	14.3−17.7	16.6
9−11 yr.	30	15.7−18.1	16.9	23	15.2−17.6	16.5	53	15.2−18.1	16.7
12−14 yr.	30	16.4−18.5	17.4	23	16.0−17.6	16.7	53	16.0−18.5	17.1
15−17 yr.	32	16.6−18.8	17.6	18	15.9−17.7	16.9	50	15.9−18.8	17.3
18−20 yr.	30	16.3−19.2	17.7	22	16.3−17.8	17.1	52	16.3−19.2	17.5
21−	360	16.3−19.5	17.8	355	15.7−18.5	17.1	715	15.7−19.5	17.5
	$\sigma = -0.52 + 0.51$			$\sigma = -0.54 + 0.39$					
	$M \pm \sigma = 17.3-18.4 = 72.1\%$			$M \pm \sigma = 16.4-17.6 = 70.2\%$					
	$M \pm 2\sigma = 16.8-18.9 = 94.2\%$			$M \pm 2\sigma = 16.0-18.1 = 95.7\%$					
TOTAL	597			545			1142		

From Haas, L. L.: Am. J. Roentgenol. 67:197 (Table V), 1952.

MEASUREMENT OF THE NORMAL SKULL

CEPHALIC INDEX *(Br × 100/L)* ON ROENTGENOGRAMS

Age	Male			Female			Total		
	n	$V_{min}-V_{max}$	M	n	$V_{min}-V_{max}$	M	n	$V_{min}-V_{max}$	M
−4 wk.	2	81.0–81.7	81.3	3	79.4–85.7	81.6	5	79.4–85.7	81.5
2–6 mo.	11	73.5–88.1	81.7	12	72.7–87.7	80.8	23	72.7–87.7	81.4
7–12 mo.	12	73.8–89.5	81.8	12	75.9–90.4	82.5	24	73.8–90.4	82.1
13–18 mo.	11	78.3–90.3	82.3	11	73.7–87.9	81.5	22	73.7–90.3	81.8
19–30 mo.	21	71.7–90.4	81.2	10	77.4–88.4	81.4	31	74.3–90.4	81.3
3–5 yr.	35	72.4–90.0	81.2	26	72.7–91.1	81.0	61	72.4–91.1	81.1
6–8 yr.	30	71.8–88.6	81.4	24	73.0–88.3	81.5	54	71.8–88.6	81.4
9–11 yr.	30	72.0–89.8	81.1	22	74.9–88.5	80.3	52	72.0–89.8	80.8
12–14 yr.	30	73.1–88.3	80.5	23	73.9–89.4	80.2	53	73.1–89.4	80.3
15–17 yr.	35	72.8–87.7	80.6	17	72.0–83.4	79.6	52	72.8–87.7	80.0
18–20 yr.	31	72.8–85.7	79.3	24	73.8–89.6	80.0	55	72.8–89.6	79.6
21–	351	71.3–89.4	79.5	354	71.0–90.4	80.0	705	71.0–90.4	79.8
	$\sigma = -3.66 + 3.87$			$\sigma = -3.87 + 3.33$					
	$M \pm \sigma = 75.9-83.4 = 65.7\%$			$M \pm \sigma = 76.1-84.2 = 66.2\%$					
	$M \pm 2\sigma = 72.2-87.3 = 96.5\%$			$M \pm 2\sigma = 72.3-88.3 = 94.0\%$					
TOTAL	599			538			1137		

From Haas, L. L.: Am. J. Roentgenol. 67:197 (Table VI), 1952.

CRANIAL INDICES IN CHILDREN

1. Technique

    a) Central ray: Anteroposterior—Directed to root of the nose with the beam angulated 15° cranially.

        Lateral—Perpendicular to the film centered over midportion of skull.

    b) Positions: Anteroposterior and lateral.

    c) Target-film distance: 80 cm.

2. Measurements

See Figure 29.

Measurements are made between the internal tables of the skull.

L = Greatest length in mm.

W = Greatest width in mm.

FIG. 29.—(Redrawn from Cronqvist,* Fig. 1.)

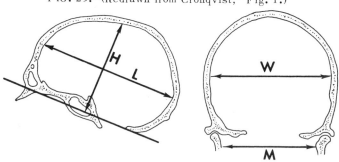

*Cronqvist, S.: Acta radiol. (Diagnosis) 7:97, 1968.

H = Greatest height in mm. measured as perpendicular distance between the vault of the skull and a line drawn from the nasion to the posterior margin of the foramen magnum.

M = Maximum distance between the inner margins of the two necks of the mandible on the anteroposterior view.

Cranial Index* $(CI) = \dfrac{L + H + W}{M} \times 10$

Age	No. of Patients	Cranial Index of Cronqvist ($\pm$2 S.D.) $\dfrac{L+H+W}{M} \times 10$	$L+H+W$ ($\pm$2 S.D.) (mm.)	Length Index ($\pm$2 S.D.) $\dfrac{L}{M} \times 10$	Width Index ($\pm$2 S.D.) $\dfrac{W}{M} \times 10$	Height Index ($\pm$2 S.D.) $\dfrac{H}{M} \times 10$	Volumetric Indices ($\pm$2 S.D.) $L \times H \times W$ (mm.³)	$\dfrac{L \times H \times W}{M^3} \times 10^3$
1st mo.	71	57 ± 5*	327 ± 26*	22 ± 2†	17 ± 2*	18 ± 2*	1,300 ± 300*	6,700 ± 1,800*
2nd and 3rd mo.	21	58 ± 4	355 ± 43	23 ± 2	17 ± 2	18 ± 2	1,600 ± 600	6,900 ± 1,300
4th through 6th mo.	22	57 ± 4	391 ± 30	22 ± 3	18 ± 2	17 ± 2	2,200 ± 500	6,600 ± 1,300
7th through 9th mo.	21	57 ± 5	421 ± 42	22 ± 3	18 ± 2	17 ± 2	2,700 ± 800	6,800 ± 1,800
10th through 12th mo.	17	56 ± 6	421 ± 36	22 ± 3	18 ± 2	16 ± 3	2,700 ± 700	6,400 ± 2,000
1 yr.	25	56 ± 6	441 ± 45	22 ± 2	18 ± 2	17 ± 2	3,120 ± 910	6,500 ± 2,300
2 yr.	20	56 ± 7	456 ± 32	22 ± 3	17 ± 2	17 ± 3	3,460 ± 730	6,400 ± 2,400
3 yr.	20	55 ± 5	470 ± 45	22 ± 3	17 ± 1	16 ± 2	3,780 ± 1,130	6,000 ± 1,900
4 yr.	21	52 ± 6	464 ± 34	20 ± 4	16 ± 2	16 ± 2	3,630 ± 790	5,300 ± 1,900
5 yr.	24	53 ± 5*	465 ± 37*	21 ± 3†	16 ± 2*	16 ± 2*	3,680 ± 880*	5,300 ± 1,600*

*The difference between the mean values for the first-month age group and the 5-year age group is statistically significant ($p < 0.001$).

†The difference between the mean values for the first-month age group and the 5-year age group is statistically significant ($p < 0.02$).

(From Austin and Gooding,‡ Table 1.)

The two most sensitive indices are the cranial index $(L + H + W/M) \times 10$ and $L + H + W$. The cranial index demonstrates an increase in head size in 90% of cases of hydrocephalus.

3. Source of Material

Ninety-six routine skull examinations and 22 normal pneumoencephalograms of children under 7 years of age (Cronqvist).

Two hundred sixty-two normal skull examinations in patients ranging in age from newborn through 5 years (Austin and Gooding).

---

*Cronqvist, S.: Acta radiol. (Diagnosis) 7:97, 1968.

‡Austin, J. H. M., and Gooding, C. A.: Radiology 99:641, 1971.

MEASUREMENT OF THE THICKNESS OF THE SKULL

1. *Technique*

   a) Central ray: To a point 1 inch anterior and 1 inch superior to external auditory meatus.

   b) Position: Lateral.

   c) Target-film distance: 70 cm. (Orley*).

   7 feet (Hansman[†]).

2. *Measurements*

   Outer table: Average thickness, 1.5 mm.*

   Inner table: Average thickness, 0.5 mm.*

   Cranial wall: Frontal region, average thickness, 5.0 mm.*

   Parietal region (measured on anteroposterior skull film) also has an average thickness of 5.0 mm. except in the region of parietal thinning.*

   Floor of skull: Average thickness, 2.0-3.0 mm.*

   Occipital (lambda[†]): See Figure 30.

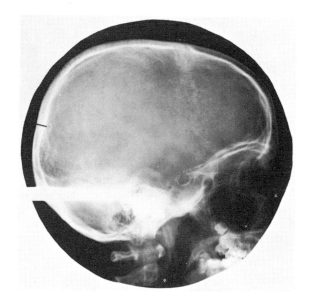

FIG. 30.—Straight line at lambda indicates site of measurement of skull thickness. (From Hansman, Fig. 1, *A*.)

*Orley, A.: *Neuroradiology* (Springfield, Ill.: Charles C Thomas, Publisher, 1949), p. 3.

[†]Hansman, C. F.: Radiology 86:87, 1966.

MEASUREMENT OF THE THICKNESS OF THE SKULL

3. Source of Material

These dimensions are from Dr. Orley's extensive experience in skull measurement. No statistics were available.

Hansman used several hundred normal individuals who have been studied by the Child Research Council of the University of Colorado.

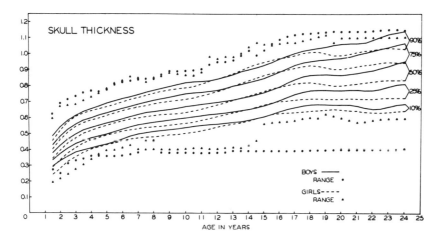

Percentile standards for skull thickness for both sexes. The thickness (cm.) on the left percentile groups is on the right. (From Hansman, Fig. 2.)

A. Vastine-Kinney Method*

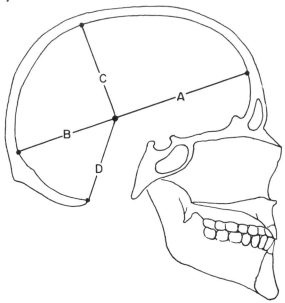

FIG. 31.—Vastine-Kinney chart for pineal position measurements.

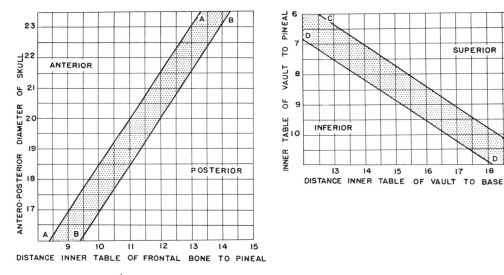

FIG. 32.—Dyke[†] modification of Vastine-Kinney chart for pineal position measurements. *Left,* normal anteroposterior variation. The measurement of *A* is plotted against the sum of *A* plus *B*. This sum is approximately equal to the greatest anteroposterior diameter of the skull. The pineal glands of normal skulls lie between *A-A* and *B-B*. *Right,* normal vertical variation. The measurement *C* is plotted against the sum of *C* plus *D*. This sum is approximately equal to the vertical diameter of the skull. The pineal glands of normal skulls lie between *C-C* and *D-D*. (From Dyke, C. G.: Am. J. Roentgenol. 23:601 (Charts II and III), 1930.)

Note: Dyke advocates moving forward 4 mm. the normal zone of Vastine and Kinney.

*Vastine, J. H., and Kinney, K. K.: Am. J. Roentgenol. 17:320, 1927.

[†]Dyke, C. G.: Am. J. Roentgenol. 23:598, 1930.

LOCALIZATION OF THE PINEAL GLAND – LATERAL PROJECTION

A. Vastine-Kinney Method

1. Technique

a) Central ray: Perpendicular to film centered over midportion of skull.
b) Position: True lateral.
c) Target-film distance: Immaterial.

2. Measurements

See Figure 31.
A = The greatest distance from the pineal body to the inner table of the frontal bone.
B = The greatest distance from the pineal body to the inner table of the occiput.
C = The greatest distance from the pineal body to the inner table of the vault.
D = The greatest distance from the pineal body to the occipital bone in the vertical direction.

3. Source of Material

This material is based on the roentgen examination of 200 skull films which were essentially negative for intracranial lesions.

B. Pawl-Walter Method[*]

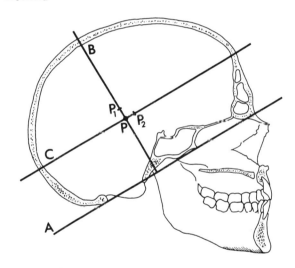

FIG. 33.–(Redrawn from Pawl and Walter, Fig. 1.)

1. Technique

a) Central ray: Perpendicular to film centered over midportion of skull.
b) Position: True lateral.
c) Target-film distance: Immaterial.

2. Measurements

See Figure 33.
Line A is drawn from nasion to lowest point of basiocciput just posterior to the opisthion.
Line B is drawn perpendicular to line A and passes through the center of the calcified pineal body (P).

---

[*]Pawl, R. P., and Walter, A. K.: Am. J. Roentgenol. 105:287, 1969.

39

B. Pawl-Walter Method

Point P_1 is one-half the distance from the baseline A to the inner table of the cranial vault.

Line C is drawn through the pineal body (P) perpendicular to line B.

Point P_2 is one-half the distance from the inner table of the frontal bone to the outer table of the occipital bone.

The pineal body (P) should lie 1 cm. below point P_1 and 1 cm. posterior to point P_2.

The range of normal is 5 mm. superior, inferior, anterior or posterior to this calculated point.

The accuracy in Pawl and Walter's series was 100% in the superoinferior dimension and 98.5% in the anteroposterior dimension.

Note:

Pawl and Walter reviewed the various methods for localization of the calcified pineal body. The Vastine-Kinney method has been included because it is familiar to many radiologists. However, the Pawl-Walter method, which does not require use of overlays and tables, has much to recommend it.

3. *Source of Material*

One hundred twenty skull examinations at Tripler Army Medical Center.

MEASUREMENT OF THE BASE OF THE SKULL
FOR BASILAR INVAGINATION

A. Chamberlain's Line*

See Figure 34. The odontoid process should not project above this (Chamberlain's) line in the normal case (S.D. ± 3.3 mm.).[†] In any individual case an odontoid process 6.6 mm. (2 S.D.) or more above this line should be considered strongly indicative of basilar impression.

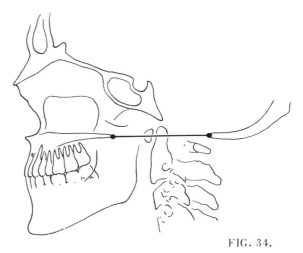

FIG. 34.

B. McRae's Line[‡]

If the line of the occipital squama is convex upward or if it lies above the line of the foramen magnum (Fig. 35[§]), basilar impression is present. In addition, a perpendicular drawn from the apex of the odontoid to the reference line should intersect it in its ventral quarter.

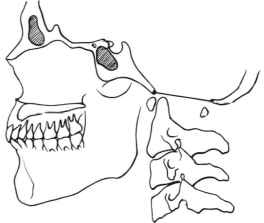

FIG. 35.—(From Hinck, Fig. 1.)

C. Method of Bull**

If angle B in Figure 36 is more than 13°, the position of the odontoid process is abnormal.

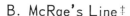

*Chamberlain, W. E.: Yale J. Biol. & Med. 11:487, 1939.

[†]Poppel, M. H., et al.: Radiology 61:639, 1953.

[‡]McRae, D. L., and Barnum, A. S.: Am. J. Roentgenol. 70:23, 1953.

[§]Hinck, V., et al.: Radiology 76:572, 1961.

**Bull, J. W., et al.: Brain 78:229, 1955.

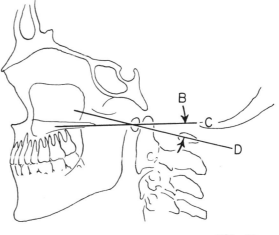

FIG. 36.

D. McGregor's Line[†]

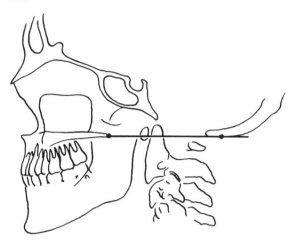

FIG. 37.

CHILDREN: BOTH SEXES (MM)[†]

Age	Mean Base Line	90% Tolerance Range
3	1.94	−0.8 - 4.7
4	2.07	−0.7 - 4.8
5	2.17	−0.6 - 4.9
6	2.24	−0.5 - 5.0
7	2.29	−0.4 - 5.1
8	2.31	−0.4 - 5.1
9	2.30	−0.4 - 5.1
10	2.27	−0.5 - 5.0
11	2.21	−0.5 - 5.0
12	2.13	−0.6 - 4.9
13	2.01	−0.7 - 4.8
14	1.88	−0.9 - 4.6
15	1.71	−1.0 - 4.5
16	1.52	−1.2 - 4.3
17	1.31	−1.4 - 4.1
18	1.07	−1.7 - 3.8

ADULTS (MM.)[†]

	Mean	S.D.	90% Tolerance Range for Normals
Male subjects	0.33	3.81	−7.4 to + 8.0 mm.
Female subjects	3.67	1.69	−2.4 to + 9.7 mm.
Male-female average difference	−3.06	....	....

[†]Hinck, V. C. and Hopkins, C. E.: Am. J. Roentgenol. 84:945, 1960.

MEASUREMENT OF THE BASE OF THE SKULL
FOR BASILAR INVAGINATION

E. Digastric Line

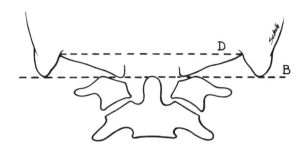

FIG. 38.—*D*, digastric line; *B*, bimastoid line.
(From Hinck, Fig. 2.)

ADULTS: MEASURED ON LAMINAGRAMS TO
ATLANTO-OCCIPITAL JOINT (MM.)[†]

	Mean	S.D.	90% Tolerance Range for Normals
Either sex	11.66	4.04	3.8 - 19.5 mm.

ADULTS: MEASURED ON LAMINAGRAMS
TO APEX OF DENS (MM.)[†]

	Mean	S.D.	90% Tolerance Range for Normals
Either sex	10.70	5.06	1.0 - 20.4 mm.

1. Technique

A. McGregor's, McRae's, and Chamberlain's lines:

   1. Central ray: Perpendicular to lateral skull.

      McGregor's—centered to C2.

      McRae's and Chamberlain's—over midportion of skull.

   2. Position: McGregor's—true lateral of cervical spine and skull. Patient sitting with head in neutral position.

      McRae's and Chamberlain's—true lateral of skull. Include upper portion of cervical spine.

   3. Target-film distance: 72 inches for McGregor's measurements.

      36 inches for Chamberlain's measurements.

[†] Hinck, V. C. and Hopkins, C. E.: Am. J. Roentgenol. 84:945, 1960.

MEASUREMENT OF THE BASE OF THE SKULL
FOR BASILAR INVAGINATION

B. Method of Bull:
As above, except that the roentgenograms must be made with the patient in the prone position and the chin in neutral position, neither flexed nor extended. Criteria do not apply in the erect position.

C. Digastric line:
   1. Central ray: To line connecting outer canthus of eye and external auditory meatus.
   2. Position: Patient supine and skull so positioned that line connecting outer canthus of eye and external auditory meatus is perpendicular to the table top.
      Anteroposterior tomograms used.
   3. Target-film distance: 40 inches.

2. *Measurements*

   A. Chamberlain's line (Fig. 34): Line from the posterior margin of the hard palate to the posterior margin of the foramen magnum.

   B. McRae's line (Fig. 35): Foramen magnum line. Line from the anterior margin of the foramen magnum (basion) to the posterior border (opisthion).

   C. Method of Bull (Fig. 36):
      C = Line drawn along plane of hard palate.
      D = Line drawn along plane of atlas.

   D. McGregor's line (Fig. 37): Line from the posterosuperior margin of the hard palate to the lowermost point on the midline occipital curve.

   E. Digastric line (Fig. 38): Line between the two digastric grooves which lie just medial to the bases of the mastoid processes.

3. *Source of Material*

The measurements of the normal position of the odontoid process in relationship to Chamberlain's line were based on a series of roentgenograms of 102 normal skulls (Poppel).

McRae's measurements were based on roentgenograms of 25 skulls.

Bull's measurements were based on roentgenograms of 120 normal skulls.

Hinck's measurements of McGregor's line were based on roentgenograms of 66 normal adult skulls and a series of 258 films taken at yearly intervals on 43 normal children, aged 3-18 years.

Hinck's measurements of the digastric line were based on skull laminagrams of 68 normal adults.

   Note:
   Studies by Hinck show that, of the various diagnostic systems to determine basilar invagination, McRae's line and the digastric line appear to be the best. McGregor's line seems to be the best measurement for use on the lateral skull film.

MEASUREMENT OF THE BASE OF THE SKULL FOR PLATYBASIA

The Basal Angle*

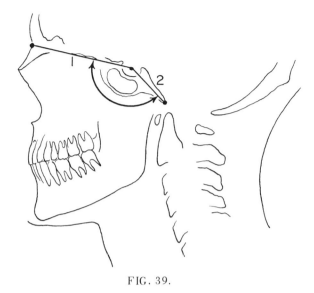

FIG. 39.

NORMAL RANGE OF THE BASAL ANGLE

Maximum ...... 152°
Minimum....... 123°
Mean .... 137°

1. *Technique*

   a) Central ray: Perpendicular to film centered over midportion of skull.

   b) Position: True lateral. Midline tomogram may be used.

   c) Target-film distance: Immaterial.

2. *Measurements*

   See Figure 39.

   1 = Line drawn from the nasion to the center of the sella turcica.

   2 = Line drawn from the center of the sella turcica to the anterior margin of the foramen magnum.

The basal angle is not a measurement of degree of impression of the base but is an index of the position of one part of the base relative to another. The base may be impressed with or without disturbance of this relationship.

3. *Source of Material*

   These measurements were based on roentgen examination in 102 normal cases.

---

*Poppel, M. H., *et al.*: Radiology 61:639, 1953.

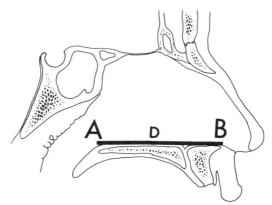

FIG. 40.—(Redrawn from Austin *et al.*, Fig. 1.)

1. *Technique*

   a) Central ray: Perpendicular to plane of film centered over the midportion of the skull.

   b) Position: Lateral

   c) Target-film distance: 40 inches

2. *Measurements*

See Figure 40.

Length of hard palate *(AB)* extends from the anterior maxillary process to posterior termination.

D = 31 mm. ± 3 mm.

   Note:

   In a newborn term infant, roentgenographic hard-palate length of 26 mm. or less is a sign of mongolism. Hard-palate length of 27 mm. or 28 mm. is indeterminate, and 29 mm. or more is within normal limits.

3. *Source of Material*

One hundred eighty-two newborn full-term infants considered to be normal at birth.

*Austin, J. H. M., *et al.:* Radiology 92:775, 1969.

NORMAL LATERAL MEASUREMENTS OF THE SELLA TURCICA*

A. Children

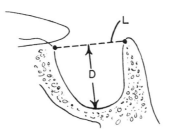

FIG. 41.

MEAN AREA OF PITUITARY FOSSA FOR GIVEN COMBINATIONS OF LENGTH AND DEPTH (BOYS)†

LENGTH IN MM.	DEPTH IN MM. *(D)*							
	3	4	5	6	7	8	9	10
5	14.5	15.0	13.0	...	...	...	...	...
6	14.1	18	19.0	...	...	...	...	...
7	17.8	20.2	25.5	35.7	36	61	...	...
8	17.2	22.3	30.0	36.8	47.4	55.9	61.0	...
9	13.0	27.3	34.2	42.0	51.4	60.2	69.9	...
10	...	31.7	38.1	46.7	55.8	65.0	74.8	87.5
11	...	29.0	41.9	51.7	60.9	69.9	81.9	85.3
12	...	45.0	47.0	57.6	64.3	72.9	81.3	92.3
13	...	...	43.9	55.2	69.7	78.1	87.3	95.0
14	...	...	61.0	66.8	73.6	81.0	87.6	97.0
15	...	...	...	58.0	71.3	90.6	103.3	97.0
16	...	...	...	...	84.0	90.0	96.7	...

†Adapted from Silverman.

FIG. 42.

MEAN AREA OF PITUITARY FOSSA FOR GIVEN COMBINATION OF LENGTH AND DEPTH (GIRLS)†

LENGTH IN MM.	DEPTH IN MM. *(D)*							
	3	4	5	6	7	8	9	10
5	14.4	16.0	22.7	42.0	43.2	39.0	...	...
6	17.4	22.0	28.2	39.1	41.9	51.1	55.0	...
7	19.8	24.7	30.5	40.4	46.8	56.6	81.7	89.0
8	21.0	28.0	35.6	43.1	52.5	61.0	74.8	...
9	...	32.0	41.0	47.9	55.2	66.7	75.7	84.9
10	...	37.5	42.7	55.9	59.1	69.4	80.6	86.2
11	...	...	49.2	60.3	68.3	78.6	85.7	92.7
12	...	...	52.0	65.8	73.2	81.4	88.4	96.2
13	...	...	...	65.4	78.6	85.4	93.8	...
14	...	...	...	...	...	...	...	...
15	...	...	...	...	...	...	...	...
16	...	...	...	...	...	...	...	...

†Adapted from Silverman.

FIG. 43.

*Silverman, F.: Am. J. Roentgenol. 78:451, 1957.

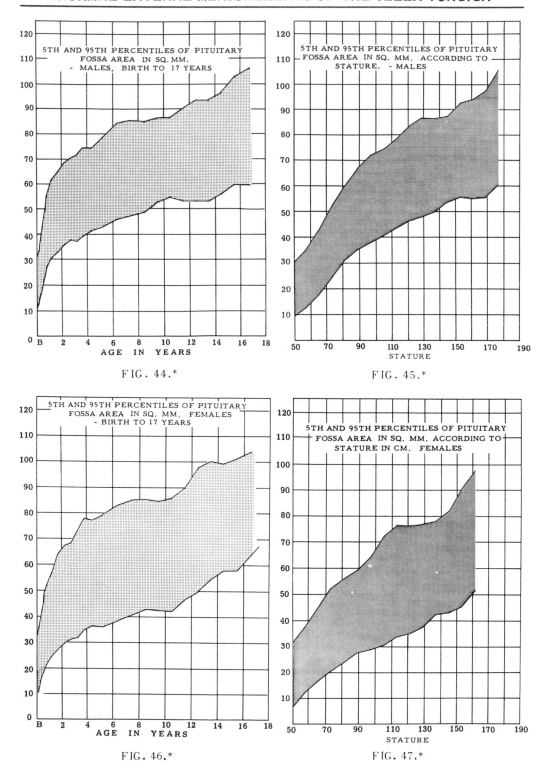

FIG. 44.*

FIG. 45.*

FIG. 46.*

FIG. 47.*

*Figures 44-47 are from Silverman, F.: Am. J. Roentgenol. 78:451 (Figs. 7-10), 1957.

NORMAL LATERAL MEASUREMENTS OF THE SELLA TURCICA

1. *Technique*
    a) Central ray: Perpendicular to plane of film centered over midportion of skull.
    b) Position: Lateral.
    c) Target-film distance: 5 feet.

2. *Measurements*

    The area of the pituitary fossa is measured with a compensating polar planimeter. Conversion to the metric system (square millimeters) is made by multiplying by the factor 6.45. The area is measured by tracing the contour from the tip of the dorsum sellae clockwise to the tuberculum sellae and then following a straight line from the tuberculum sellae back to the point of origin. In cases where the tip of the dorsum sellae could be visualized through the clinoid processes, the line of reference is drawn to the visual boundaries of the dorsum sellae, disregarding the superimposition of the clinoid processes.

    The length (L, Fig. 41) is the distance from the dorsum sellae to the tuberculum sellae corresponding to the position of the diaphragmatic sellae. The depth is a perpendicular line dropped to the deepest point (D, Fig. 41). In the absence of a compensating polar planimeter, the measurements of the pituitary fossa are obtained as outlined. By referring to the table for the appropriate sex (Fig. 42 or 43) the mean area is observed. This mean figure is located on graphs where the area is plotted against age (Figs. 44 and 46), or on graphs where the area is plotted against height (Figs. 45 and 47). The height of the subject is probably a better standard for evaluation of pituitary fossa area than age. These graphs indicate the position of the pituitary fossa with respect to pituitary fossae from a group of normal children of the same age and the same height. A value for the area obtained from Figure 42 or 43 which lies outside the 5th and 95th percentiles would have real significance with respect to indicating a deviation from the normal.

    > *Note:*
    > The significance of the small sella turcica is open to question in the light of Di Chiro's work on the small sella turcica. See page 51.

3. *Source of Material*

    These data have been based on measurements of the pituitary fossa seen in lateral roentgenograms of the skull on 2,137 films from 168 boys, and on 1,899 films from 152 girls, between the ages of 1 month and 18 years. The children were participants in the longitudinal growth study of the Fels Research Institute.

NORMAL LATERAL MEASUREMENTS OF THE SELLA TURCICA*

B. Adults

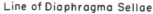

Line of Diaphragma Sellae

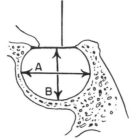

FIG. 48.

NORMAL RANGE OF MEASUREMENTS

	MAX.	MIN.	AV.
A (anteroposterior diameter, in mm.)	16	5	10.6
B (depth, in mm.)	12	4	8.1

1. Technique

a) Central ray: 2.5 cm. in front and 1.9 cm. above the external auditory meatus.

b) Position: True lateral. Essential that sagittal plane of the head be parallel with the film and perpendicular to the central ray.

c) Target-film distance: 36 inches.

2. Measurements

See Figure 48.

A = Greatest anteroposterior diameter.

B = Greatest depth.

3. Source of Material

These measurements were based on a study of 500 roentgenograms which had been reported as roentgenologically negative. The dimensions coincide with those obtained by direct measurement of anatomic specimens by Camp.

THE SELLAR-CRANIAL INDEX**

1. Technique

Same as used for lateral measurements of the sella turcica.

2. Measurements

$$\text{Index} = \frac{\text{Greatest anteroposterior diameter of sella}}{\text{Maximum length between inner table of frontal bone and inner table of occipital bone}} \times 100.$$

Index in 200 normal subjects: 26% had index of 5, 53% had index of 6, 21% had index of 7,

3. Source of Material

Two hundred normal subjects.

*Camp, J. D.: Radiology 1:65, 1923.

**Martinez-Farinas, L. O.: Radiology 88:264, 1967.

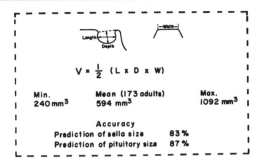

FIG. 49.—The volume of the sella
turcica. (From Di Chiro and Nelsen.*)

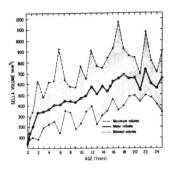

FIG. 50.—Sellar volumes of 347
"normal" controls. (From Fisher
and Di Chiro, Fig. 3.†)

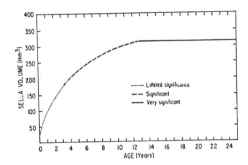

FIG. 51.—Minimal expected normal
sellar volumes. (From Fisher and
Di Chiro, Fig. 4.†)

1. *Technique*
   a) Central ray: Posteroanterior — to glabella; lateral — to a point 1 inch anterior
   and 1 inch superior to external auditory meatus.
   b) Positions: Posteroanterior; lateral.
   c) Target-film distance: 36 inches.

2. *Measurements*

   See Figures 49, 50 and 51.

3. *Source of Material*

   These measurements were based on 60 cases* in a series, later extended to 80
   cases,† in which the sellar volume calculated from posteroanterior and lateral
   roentgenograms was compared with the volume determined by filling the sella turcica
   with dentist's wax. The method was then tested on 347 "normals."†

   Di Chiro has pointed out that the sellar size cannot be reliably estimated from the
   lateral roentgenogram alone. Knowing the three linear dimensions of the sella, it is
   possible to state pituitary gland size and sellar size so that 90% of the cases will
   be accurate within approximately 30%. The "best estimate" of pituitary gland volume
   from pituitary fossa measurements requires the use of regression analysis.‡

*Di Chiro, G., and Nelsen, K. B.: Am. J. Roentgenol. 87:989, 1962.

†Fisher, R. L., and Di Chiro, G.: Am. J. Roentgenol. 91:996, 1964.

‡McLachlan. M. S. F.; Williams, E. D.; Fortt, R. W.; and Doyle, F. H.: Brit. J. Radiol.
41:323, 1968.

MEASUREMENT OF THE OPTIC FORAMINA

Right   Left

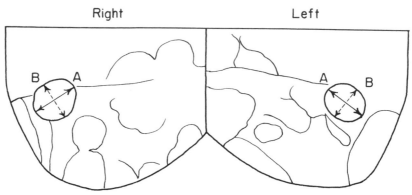

FIG. 52.

MEASUREMENTS CORRECTED FOR ROENTGENOGRAPHIC DISTORTION*

	A (IN MM.)			B (IN MM.)		
	Max.	Min.	Av.	Max.	Min.	Av.
Right side	5.3	3.5	4.26	5.6	3.0	4.33
Left side	5.6	3.5	4.49	5.5	3.5	4.30

Newborn: Average maximum diameter is 4 mm.[†] Age 6 months: Average maximum diameter is 5 mm. Optic foramina reach adult size at about 5 years.

1. *Technique*

    a) Central ray: Perpendicular to film passing through center of orbit being examined. Pfeiffer method:[†] 37° to sagittal plane and 30° to canthomeatal plane.

    b) Position: Rotate the head 53° from the true frontal position toward the orbit under study, so that the supraorbital ridge and zygomatic arch rest firmly on the plate. Pfeiffer method[†] requires V-shaped cassette tunnel to support patient's head.

    c) Target-film distance: Pfeiffer method:[†] 25 inches. Immaterial for adult measurements.

2. *Measurements*

    See Figure 52.

    A = Line from the superomesial margin of the canal to the inferolateral extremity at an angle of 45°.

    B = Line from the superolateral edge to the inferomesial border at a right angle to A.

3. *Source of Material*

    These measurements were based on a radiographic study of 80 normal skulls and have been corrected for radiographic distortion.

---

*Goalwin, H. A.: Am. J. Roentgenol. 13:480, 1925; also Young, B. R.: *The Skull, Sinuses, Mastoids: A Handbook of Roentgen Diagnosis* (Chicago: Year Book Medical Publishers, Inc., 1948).

[†]Evans, R. A., *et al.*: Radiol. Clin. North America 1:459, 1963. Contains description of Pfeiffer method.

LOCALIZATION OF INTRAOCULAR FOREIGN BODIES

A. Sweet's Method*

In 1898 Sweet described his method and first apparatus. In 1909 he described his improved apparatus.* It is remarkable that after 60 years this improved model is still one of the best and most popular methods of localization.

A lead ball-indicator is used to orientate the center of the cornea, and by means of a mirror and a telescope this indicator is adjusted exactly 1 cm. away from the center of the cornea and in the optical axis. Two semilateral radiograms are then taken on one film—the second exposure with a caudal displacement of the tube.

In the Sweet apparatus the tube, ball-indicator and film-holder are all on a movable stage, in constant relation to one another. The tube-film distance and the angle of the central ray with the optical axis are both constant, so that the same indicator serves for both exposures. For illustrations of equipment and for charts See Shanks and Kerley,[†] Figs. 581-585, pp. 556-560.

The optical axis is fixed by the sound eye—an advantage, since often the damaged eye is sightless.

The localization is carried out in the following steps:

a) Place the patient supine with the film on the side of the head nearest the injured eye.

b) Adjust the ball-indicator vertically 1 cm. above the center of the cornea.

c) Take the first radiogram with the tube in the middle position of the scale (the central ray at right angles to the long axis of the patient's body and passing through the center of the iris of the damaged eye).

d) Take the second picture with the tube displaced to the end of the scale nearest the feet.

e) Superimpose the film on the key-plate and read the co-ordinates of the two shadows of the foreign body.

f) Mark these co-ordinates on the chart; their intersections mark the position of the foreign body within or without the eye.

1. *Method of Adjustment of Indicator-ball.*—The operator looks through the aperture in the mirror and aligns the ball-indicator over the center of the cornea of the injured eye. This ensures that the optical axis of that eye is parallel to the film. The ball is then adjusted to a distance 1 cm. from the surface of the center of the cornea, by looking through the telescope and bringing the image in the telescope mirror of the cross-wire into a position tangential to that of the center of the cornea. A small lamp gives the necessary illumination. The variation of distance, due to parallactic error, is stated to be only 0.1 mm.

2. *The Exposures.*—The eyes must remain immobile throughout the two exposures. To facilitate this, both are made on different portions of one film.

   First Exposure: The film is placed *in situ* and the lead shutters are opened to leave the center part of the film unprotected. The tube is set at zero on the scale and the first exposure is made.

   Second Exposure: The tube is moved down to the limit caudally, and the upper (cephalic) lead shutter is moved down to protect the center of the film and lay bare the cephalic portion. The second exposure is then made, one 50% heavier being given.

3. *Charting the Radiogram.*—Place the developed film with its tube side against the key-plate and move it till the two shadows of the indicator-ball coincide with the balls on the key-plate, which is a graph provided with the apparatus. The key-plate is not shown here.

---

*Sweet, W. M.: Arch. Ophth. 38:623, 1909.

[†]Shanks, S. C., and Kerley, P.: *A Text-Book of X-Ray Diagnosis*. (Philadelphia: W. B. Saunders Co., 1969), vol. 1, pp. 555-560.

C or *D* Reading: The film and key are illuminated and the distance of the shadow of the foreign body to the right *(C)* or left *(D)* of the indicator-ball is noted and transferred to the corresponding lines of the *C* or *D* section of the final chart, on the right or left side, according to which eye is being examined.

E Reading: Without moving the film the *E* reading (the depth of the foreign body from the tangent of the center of the cornea) is taken and plotted on the *E* section of the chart.

A or *B* Reading: To take this (the horizontal distance from the vertical zero line in the second radiogram) the shadow of the indicator-ball in the second (oblique) radiogram is made to coincide with the right or left indicator-ball on the key-plate.

The *A* (or *B*) co-ordinate that crosses the shadow of the foreign body is read and plotted on *A* or *B* lines in the chart. (The vertical co-ordinate, *E*, should be the same in both readings.) If the tube was accurately centered in its holder, the shadow of the indicator-ball in the radiogram will coincide with those on the key-plate and it will then not be necessary to reset the radiogram to read the position of the *A* and *B* co-ordinates.

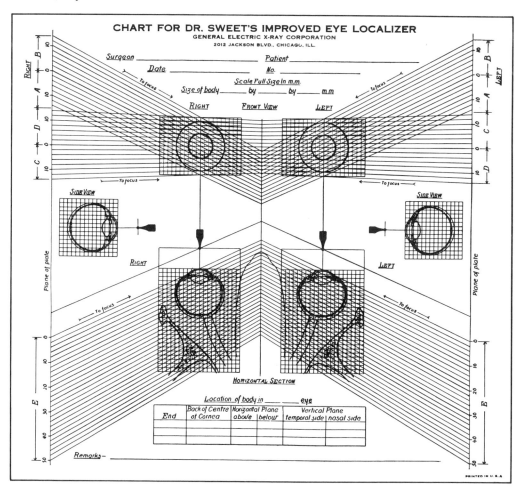

4. *Interpretation of the Chart.*—*(a)* The intersection of the plotted lines *A* or *B*, and *C* or *D* gives the position of the foreign body from the front; *i.e.*, above or below the center of the cornea and to the nasal or temporal side. *(b)* The intersection of a vertical abscissa from the point with the *E* reading gives the depth of the foreign body from the cornea. *(c)* The situation of the foreign body in the side view is determined by plotting in the appropriate lateral diagram its measured depth from

the cornea and its distance above or below the axis of the globe. The intersection of the two gives the site of the foreign body. Note, however, that the shadow of the foreign body may be within the ocular contour in three planes and yet be extraocular.

B. Contact Lens Method [†]

A plastic contact lens containing four radiopaque marker dots is placed on the cornea. This is used to measure magnification. Radiographs are made in the anteroposterior and lateral positions. Measurements are made on these films for the localization of the foreign body. Measurements corrected for distortion are plotted on a chart.

Equipment for the contact-lens method is being manufactured.

[†]Pfeiffer, R. L.: Am. J. Roentgenol. 44:558, 1940.

DEVELOPMENT OF THE PARANASAL SINUSES*

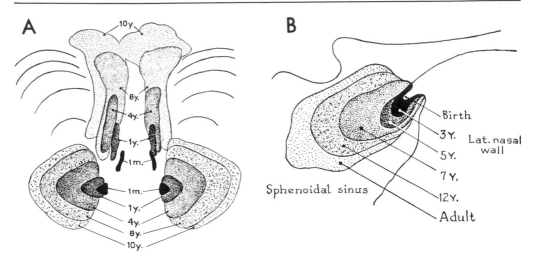

FIG. 53.—*A*, composite drawing showing the changes in size and shape of the maxillary and frontal sinuses in one individual during infancy and childhood (*m*, month; *y*, year). *B*, diagram illustrating the postnatal growth of the sphenoid sinus from birth to maturity. (From Caffey, Fig. 126 [*A* redrawn from Maresh, M. M.: Am. J. Dis. Child. 60:55, 1940; *B* redrawn from Scammon in *Abt's Pediatrics*].)

A. Frontal and Maxillary Sinuses

1. Technique

    a) Central ray: Perpendicular to table top.
    b) Position: Posteroanterior. Head on 23° board.
    c) Target-film distance: 28 inches.

2. Measurements. None.

3. Source of Material

    Figure 53, *A*, was made from tracings of roentgenograms of 100 children who were examined periodically from birth to maturity.

B. Sphenoid Sinus

1. Technique

    a) Central ray: Perpendicular to table top.
    b) Position: True lateral.
    c) Target-film distance: Irrelevant.

2. Measurements. None.

3. Source of Material

Maresh studied the frontal, ethmoid, and maxillary sinuses on routine anteroposterior roentgenograms of 100 children who were being examined from birth to maturity by the Child Research Council.

    For studies on the sphenoid sinus, see the work of Schaeffer, J. P.: Pennsylvania M. J. 39:395, 1936. Schaeffer measured 3,000 sphenoid sinus specimens.

---

*Caffey, J.: *Pediatric X-Ray Diagnosis* (3d ed.; Chicago: Year Book Publishers, Inc., 1956), pp. 93-101.

MEASUREMENT OF THE MAXILLARY, FRONTAL, AND SPHENOID SINUSES*

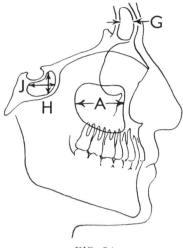

FIG. 54.

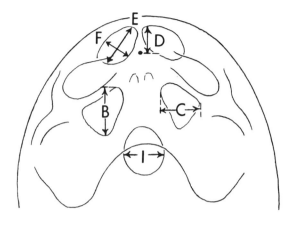

FIG. 55.

MAXILLARY SINUSES (IN MM.)

AGE	A	B	C	
Newborn	7.0-8.0	4.0-6.0	3.0-4.0	
9 mo.	11.0-14.0	5.0-5.0	5.0-5.5	
1 yr.	14.0-16.0	6.0-6.5	5.0-6.0	
2 yr.	21.0-22.0	10.0-11.0	8.0-9.0	
3 yr.	22.0-23.0	11.0-12.0	9.0-10.0	
6 yr.	27.0-28.0	16.0-17.0	16.0-17.0	
10 yr.	30.0-31.0	17.5-18.0	19.0-20.0	
15 yr.	31.0-32.0	18.0-20.0	19.0-20.0	
18 yr.	31.0-33.0	20.0-21.0	19.0-21.0	

FRONTAL SINUSES (IN MM.)

AGE	D	E	F	G
6-12 mo.	2.0	2.0	2.0	3.5
1-2 yr.	1.8	5.0	2.5	4.5
3-4 yr.	2.5	7.0	4.0	5.5
7-8 yr.	9.5	13.0	10.0	8.5
10-11 yr.	12.5	16.0	10.0	9.0
13-14 yr.	12.0	16.0	9.5	10.0
17-18 yr.	15.0	18.0	20.0	16.0
19-20 yr.	28.0	26.0	26.0	17.0

*Schaeffer, J. P.: Pennsylvania M. J. 39:395, 1936.

MEASUREMENT OF THE MAXILLARY, FRONTAL, AND SPHENOID SINUSES

SPHENOID SINUSES (IN MM.)

AGE	SIDE	H	I	J
1 yr.	R	2.5	2.5	1.5
	L	2.5	2.5	1.5
2 yr.	R	4.0	3.5	2.2
	L	4.0	3.5	2.2
5 yr.	R	7.0	6.5	4.5
	L	6.5	6.8	4.7
9 yr.	R	15.0	12.0	10.0
	L	14.5	11.5	11.0
14 yr.	R	14.0	9.0	12.0
	L	15.0	14.0	7.0

1. Technique

The charted measurements are actual anatomic dimensions.

2. Measurements

See Figures 54 and 55 and to the tables below the figures.

A = Anteroposterior dimension of maxillary sinus.
B = Vertical height of maxillary sinus.
C = Width of maxillary sinus.
D = Distance of cupola of frontal sinus above nasion.
E = Height of frontal sinus.
F = Width of frontal sinus.
G = Length of frontal sinus.
H = Height of sphenoid sinus.
I = Width of sphenoid sinus.
J = Length of sphenoid sinus.

3. Source of Material

These measurements represent actual anatomic measurements based on a study of more than 3,000 specimens.

MEASUREMENT OF PARANASAL SINUS MUCOUS MEMBRANE THICKNESS*

1. *Technique*

   a) Central ray: Caldwell—To nasion.

   Waters—To anterior nasal spine.

   Anteroposterior basal—Perpendicular to base of skull and to mid-point of inferior orbitomeatal line on median plane.

   b) Position: Caldwell projection.

   Waters projection.

   Anteroposterior basal.

   c) Target-film distance: The measurements given below are anatomic thicknesses. Therefore, if sinus films are taken at a target-film distance of 36 inches, a correction should be made to a 72 inch target-film distance.

2. *Measurements*

   Frontal sinus: Caldwell projection.
   0.06 - 0.5 mm.

   Ethmoid sinus: Caldwell projection.
   0.08 - 0.45 mm.

   Sphenoid sinus: Anteroposterior basal projection.
   0.07 - 0.6 mm.

   Maxillary sinus: Waters projection.
   Medial wall, 0.2 - 1.2 mm.
   Lateral wall, 0.1 - 0.5 mm.

   Average thickness in health varies from 0.6 mm. for the medial wall of the maxillary sinus to 0.1 mm. for the ethmoid, sphenoid, and frontal sinuses. Thicknesses varying from 2.0 to 6.0 mm. are found in pathologic states.

3. *Source of Material*

   Measurements were made of 3,000 sinus specimens. The measurements given above are anatomic thicknesses.

---

*Schaeffer, J. P.: Pennsylvania M. J. 39:395, 1936.

MEASUREMENT OF INTERORBITAL DISTANCE*

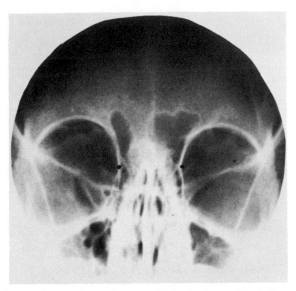

FIG. 56.—Black dots indicate the points at which the interorbital distance is measured. (From Hansman, Fig. 1, *B*.)

1. *Technique*

   a) Central ray: To anterior nasal spine.
   b) Position: Sinus film, using an angle board with nose and forehead touching the cassette and the tube in a vertical position.
   c) Target-film distance: 28 inches.

2. *Measurements*

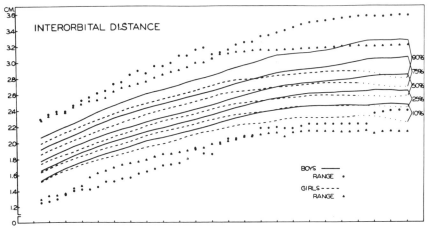

Percentile standards for measurement of interorbital distance for both sexes. Distance (cm.) on the left and percentile scale on the right. (From Hansman, Fig. 2.)

3. *Source of Material*

   Hansman used several hundred normal individuals who have been studied by the Child Research Council, University of Colorado.

*Hansman, C. F.: Radiology 86:87, 1966.

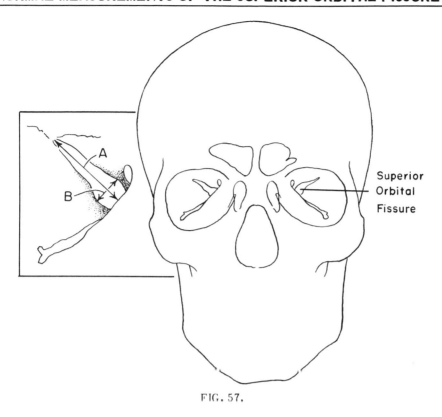

FIG. 57.

MEASUREMENTS OF ANATOMIC SPECIMENS

A (length) .... 15 mm. (av.)
B (maximal width) .... 5 mm. (av.)

1. *Technique*

   a) Central ray: Directed toward external occipital protuberance and angulated 15° toward the feet.

   b) Position: Posteroanterior. Head placed with forehead and nose touching table top.

   c) Target-film distance: 40 inches.

2. *Measurements*

   See Figure 57.

   A = Greatest length.
   B = Maximum width.

   Normal sphenoid fissures showed asymmetric development, compared with the opposite side, in 9% of cases measured.

3. *Source of Material*

   These measurements were based on a study of 157 anatomic specimens.

---

*Kornblum, K., and Kennedy, G. R.: Am. J. Roentgenol. 47:845, 1942.

MEASUREMENT OF THE INTERNAL AUDITORY CANAL*

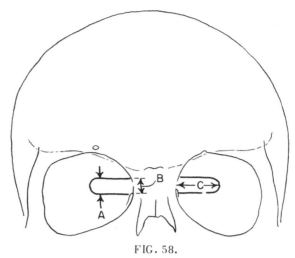

FIG. 58.

1. *Technique*

   a) Central ray: To glabella.
   b) Position: Anteroposterior, with the head placed at such an angle that the shadow of the petrous pyramids is cast through the orbits.
   c) Target-film distance: 84 inches.

2. *Measurements*

   See Figure 58.

       A = Canal diameter = Greatest diameter of canal.
           Av., 5.2 mm.; max., 11 mm.; min., 2.5 mm.
       B = Open or medial end of canal.
           Av. width, 6.2 mm.
       C = Length of canal from the superior part of the area cribosa to the most mesial point on the concave margin of the posterior wall of the canal.
           Av., 7.9 mm.; max., 16 mm.; min., 3 mm.

From the study of 100 bones, Camp and Cilley found that in approximately 30% of the bones the right and left canals differed by less than 1 mm. in depth and 0.5 mm. in diameter.

The thin posterior wall of the internal meatus is usually destroyed to some extent by a tumor mass, which causes dilation of the porus acusticus with consequent shortening of the canal.

3. *Source of Material*

The measurements were based on the examination of 509 individual bones. The bones were normal specimens obtained at necropsy, and in no instance was there evidence of erosion or other abnormality.

*Camp, J. D., and Cilley, E. I. L.: Am. J. Roentgenol. 41:713, 1939.

MEASUREMENT OF FORAMINA IN THE SKULL BASE*

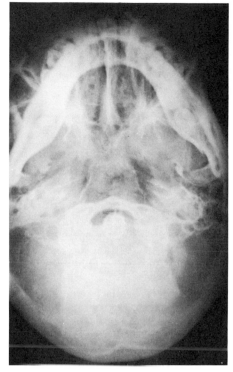

FIG. 59.

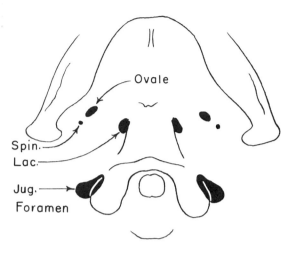

FIG. 60.

1. Technique

a) Central ray: Perpendicular to inferior orbitomeatal line at angle of mandible.

b) Position: Basal (anteroposterior).

c) Target-film distance: 70 cm.

2. Measurements

See Figures 59 and 60.

Foramen spinosum: Contains middle meningeal vessels.
Average length of short diameter, 2 mm.
Minimum length, 1 mm.
Maximum length, 3.5 mm.
The shape of the canal on radiographic projection is oval. The round artery fills the foramen from side to side in the short diameter.
In 97% of the cases the right and left foramen are almost equal in size.

Foramen ovale: Contains mandibular nerve and accessory meningeal artery.
Length, 5-11 mm.
Width, 3-7 mm.

Foramen lacerum (carotid canal): Contains internal carotid artery.
Average diameter, 6.4 mm.
Minimum diameter, 5.5 mm.
Maximum diameter, 7.0 mm.
Measurements are taken in the lateral portion of the canal corresponding to its narrowest point.

*Orley, A.: *Neuroradiology* (Springfield, Ill.: Charles C Thomas, Publisher, 1949), p. 45.

MEASUREMENT OF FORAMINA IN THE SKULL BASE

Jugular foramen: Consists of three portions:

Lateral portion: Corresponds to jugular vein.
  Right side average, 12.9 × 8.6 mm.
  Left side average, 11.6 × 7.6 mm.
  Minimum, 6 × 7 mm.
  Maximum, 12 × 16 mm.
Medial portion:
  Minimum, 2 × 4 mm.
  Maximum, 3 × 5 mm.
Intermediate portion: Contains 9th, 10th, and 11th cranial nerves.
  Minimum, 3 × 5 mm.
  Maximum, 4 × 6 mm.

3. *Source of Material*

These measurements are from Orley's extensive experience in skull measurement. No statistics were available.

DEVELOPMENT OF THE TEETH*

APPROXIMATE PERIODS OF ERUPTION†
(See also Figure 61)

DECIDUOUS TEETH

TEETH	ERUPTION OCCURS	SHEDDING BEGINS
Medial incisors	6-8 mo.	7th yr.
Lateral incisors	7-12 mo.	8th yr.
First molars	14-15 mo.	10th yr.
Canines	18-19 mo.	10th yr.
Second molars	20-24 mo.	11th-12th yr.

PERMANENT TEETH

TEETH	YEAR ERUPTION OCCURS	
	Girls	Boys
First molars	6.0	6.5
Medial incisors	6.5	7.0
Lateral incisors	8.0	8.5
First premolars	9.0	10.0
Second premolars	10.0	11.0
Canines	11.0	11.5
Second molars	11.5	12.0
Third molars	17-25	17-25

*Schour, I., and Poncher, H.; copyright 1940 and 1945 by Mead Johnson & Company.

†Pendergrass, E. P.; Schaeffer, J. P.; and Hodes, P.: *The Head and Neck in Roentgen Diagnosis*, Vol. I (Springfield, Ill.: Charles C Thomas, Publisher, 1956), p. 442.

DEVELOPMENT OF THE TEETH

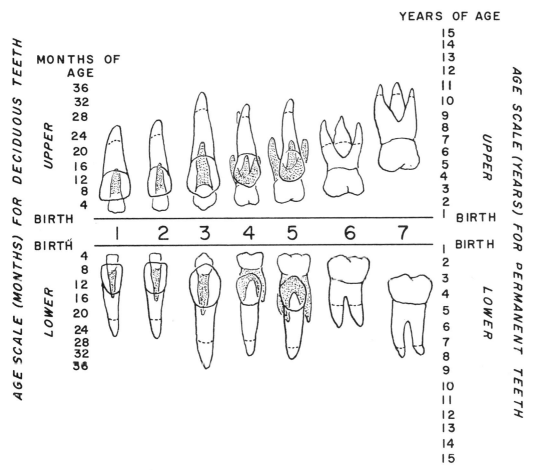

FIG. 61.—Schematic representation of the velocity of calcification and eruption of the teeth. The position of the biting edge of the crowns in the age scale indicates the age at which calcification of each tooth begins. Dotted lines on the roots signify the age at which each tooth erupts and its approximate size at that time. The position of the ends of the roots on the age scale measures the age at which calcification of each tooth is completed. The third permanent molar is not shown because of its great normal developmental variation. It usually begins to calcify between age 7 and 10, erupts between age 17 and 21, and completes calcification between age 18 and 25. Deciduous teeth are shaded; permanent teeth are unshaded. (Redrawn from Schour and Poncher.)

B. Skeletal Maturation

A. Method of Sontag, Snell, and Anderson*

LIST OF CENTERS (TOTAL, 67)

Shoulder .....Coracoid process
Humerus .....Proximal medial epiphysis
 Proximal lateral epiphysis
 Capitellum
 Medial epicondyle
Radius ....Proximal epiphysis
 Distal epiphysis
Hand.........Capitatum
 Hamatum
 Triquetrum
 Lunate
 Navicula
 Greater multiangular bone
 Lesser multiangular bone
 5 distal phalangeal epiphyses
 4 middle phalangeal epiphyses
 5 proximal phalangeal epiphyses
 5 metacarpal epiphyses

Femur ....Proximal epiphysis
 Greater trochanter
 Distal epiphysis
Knee..........Patella
Tibia ....Proximal epiphysis
 Distal epiphysis
Fibula ....Proximal epiphysis
 Distal epiphysis
Foot...........Cuboid
 First cuneiform
 Second cuneiform
 Third cuneiform
 Navicula
 Epiphysis of calcaneus
 5 distal phalangeal epiphyses
 4 middle phalangeal epiphyses
 5 proximal phalangeal epiphyses
 5 metatarsal epiphyses

MEAN TOTAL NUMBER OF CENTERS ON THE LEFT SIDE OF BODY OSSIFIED AT GIVEN AGE LEVELS

AGE (in Mo.)	BOYS		GIRLS	
	Mean No.	S.D.	Mean No.	S.D.
1..........................	4.11	1.41	4.58	1.76
3..........................	6.63	1.86	7.78	2.16
6..........................	9.61	1.95	11.44	2.53
9..........................	11.88	2.66	15.36	4.92
12..........................	13.96	3.96	22.40	6.93
18..........................	19.27	6.61	34.10	8.44
24..........................	29.21	8.10	43.44	6.65
30..........................	37.59	7.40	48.91	6.50
36..........................	43.42	5.34	52.73	5.48
42..........................	47.06	5.26	56.61	3.98
48..........................	51.24	4.59	57.94	3.91
54..........................	53.94	4.35	59.89	3.36
60..........................	56.24	4.07	61.52	2.69

*Sontag, L. W.; Snell, D.; and Anderson, M.: Rate of appearance of ossification centers from birth to age five years, Am. J. Dis. Child. 58:949, 1939.

SKELETAL MATURATION

A. Method of Sontag, Snell, and Anderson

1. *Technique*

Roentgenograms are taken of the following areas of the left side of the body: shoulder, elbow, wrist and hand, hip, knee (anteroposterior; lateral after 24 months), ankle and foot (anteroposterior; lateral after 48 months).

2. *Measurements*

The total number of ossification centers in the left half of the body is counted. A center is counted as soon as it casts a small shadow on the roentgenogram.

3. *Source of Material*

These data have been taken from roentgenograms made at regular intervals of all the bones and joints of the left upper and lower extremities of 149 normal children during their first 5 years of life. The children came from the rural and metropolitan area near Yellow Springs, Ohio. There were 75 boys and 74 girls, and they represented a fair economic cross-section. Three Negro children (1 boy and 2 girls) were included.

B. Method of Girdany and Golden*

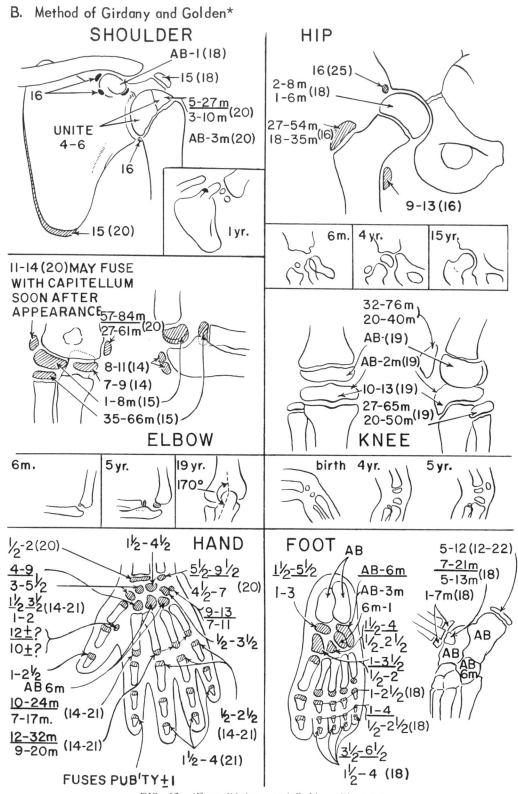

FIG. 62.—(From Girdany and Golden, Chart I.)

*Girdany, B. R., and Golden, R.: Am. J. Roentgenol. 68:922, 1952.

B. Method of Girdany and Golden

1. Technique

Conventional technique for each body part.

2. Measurements

The numbers on Figures 62 and 63 indicate the range from the 10th to the 90th percentile in appearance time of centers of ossification, obtained from the studies on bone growth available in 1950. Statistically significant studies of the time of appearance of ossification centers have been made of relatively few portions of the skeleton after the 6th year of life. Figures followed by *m* mean months; otherwise all numbers indicate years. Where two sets of numbers are given for one center of ossification, the upper figures refer to males and the lower figures refer to females. A single set of figures applies to both sexes. *AB* indicates that the ossification center is visible at birth. Figures in parentheses give approximate time of fusion.

3. Source of Material

The figures giving the range of time of appearance of the most important ossification centers have been taken from multiple sources, including:

Scammon, R. E., in *Morris' Human Anatomy*, by Morris, H.; ed. by Schaeffer, J. P. (11th ed.; Philadelphia: Blakiston Company, 1953), p. 11.

Vogt, E. C., and Vickers, V. S.: Radiology 31:441, 1938.

Milman, D. H., and Bakwin, H.: J. Pediat., 36:617, 1950.

Buehl, C. C., and Pyle, S. I.: J. Pediat. 21:331, 1942.

Ruckensteiner, E.: *Die normale Entwicklung des Knochensystems im Roentgenbilg* (Leipzig: Georg Thieme, 1931).

Bailey, W.: Am. J. Roentgenol. 42:85, 1939.

B. Method of Girdany and Golden

VERTEBRA

OSSIFY FROM 3 PRIMARY CENTERS AND 9 SECONDARY CENTERS — ANY OF THESE
SECONDARY CENTERS, EXCEPT FOR ANNULAR EPIPHYSES, MAY FAIL TO FUSE.

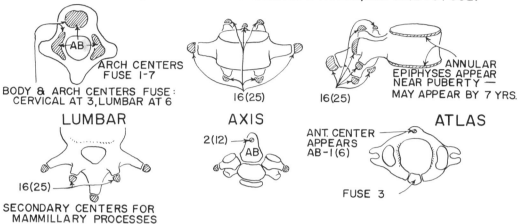

BODY & ARCH CENTERS FUSE:
CERVICAL AT 3, LUMBAR AT 6

ARCH CENTERS
FUSE 1-7

16(25)   16(25)

ANNULAR
EPIPHYSES APPEAR
NEAR PUBERTY —
MAY APPEAR BY 7 YRS.

LUMBAR   **AXIS**   **ATLAS**

2(12) — AB

ANT. CENTER
APPEARS
AB-1(6)

16(25) —

SECONDARY CENTERS FOR
MAMMILLARY PROCESSES

FUSE 3

SACRUM & COCCYX

LOWER SACRAL BODIES FUSE
AT 18 ··· ALL FUSE BY 30

INNOMINATE

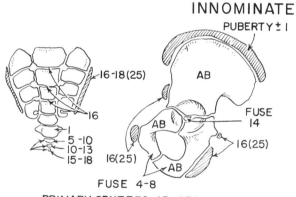

PUBERTY ± 1

— 16-18(25)

AB

— 16

FUSE
14

I
5-10
10-13
15-18

16(25)

AB

16(25)

AB

FUSE 4-8

PRIMARY CENTERS AB, SECONDARY
CENTERS APPEAR NEAR PUBERTY,
FUSE 16-30 YRS. — OCCASIONAL CENTERS
AT PUBIC TUBERCLE, ANGLE, & CREST

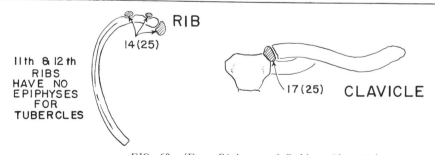

RIB

14(25)

11th & 12th
RIBS
HAVE NO
EPIPHYSES
FOR
TUBERCLES

17(25)   **CLAVICLE**

FIG. 63.—(From Girdany and Golden, Chart II.)

C. Method of Francis

*Birth to 5 Years**

DATES OF APPEARANCE OF CENTERS OF OSSIFICATION
BIRTH TO 5 YRS. OF AGE – WHITE FEMALES

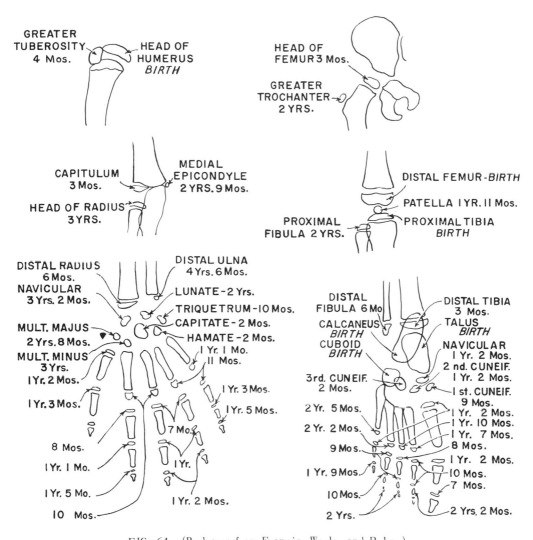

FIG. 64.–(Redrawn from Francis, Werle, and Behm.)

*Francis, C. C.; Werle, P. P.; and Behm, A.: Am. J. Phys. Anthropol. 24:273, 1939.

C. Method of Francis*

DATES OF APPEARANCE OF CENTERS OF OSSIFICATION
BIRTH TO 5 YRS OF AGE, WHITE MALES

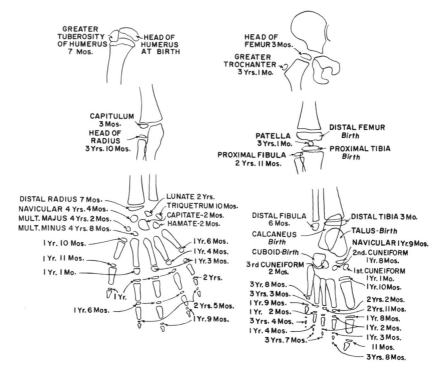

FIG. 65.—(Redrawn from Francis, Werle, and Behm.[†])

OSSIFICATION AND FUSION OF THE STERNUM[‡]

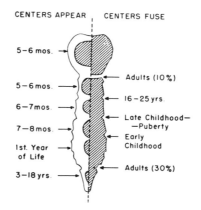

FIG. 66.—(From Currarino and Silverman, Fig. 8.)

*Francis, C.C.: Am. J. Phys. Anthropol. 27:127, 1940.

†Francis, C.C.; Werle, P.P.; and Behm, A.: Am. J. Phys. Anthropol. 24:273, 1939.

‡Currarino, G., and Silverman, F.N.: Radiology 70:532, 1958.

SKELETAL MATURATION

C. Method of Francis*

Female: 6 - 15 Years

Age	Center
6 years 8 months	Olecranon
6 years 10 months	Epiphysis of talus
7 years 1 month	Pisiform
7 years 2 months	Trochlea of humerus
7 years 7 months	Lesser troch. femur
8 years 2 months	Sesamoids of flex. hall. brevis
8 years 3 months	Hum. lat. epicondyle
8 years 7 months	5 metat. prox.
9 years 0 months	Tib. tubercle
9 years 3 months	Ant. inf. iliac spine*
9 years 4 months	Sesamoid of flex. poll. brevis
10 years 10 months	Tubercle, rib 1
11 years 3 months	Coracoid angle
11 years 4 months	Trans. proc. T 1; Acromion
12 years 0 months	Iliac crest
13 years 2 months	Ischial tuber.*
14 years 6 months	Med. clav.

* Provisional.

FIG. 67.—(Adapted from Francis.)

Male: 5-15 Years

Age	Center
5 years 2 months	Hum. med. epicondyle
5 years 6 months	Ulna, dist.
6 years 2 months	Epiphysis of calcaneus
8 years 0 months	Epiphysis of talus
8 years 4 months	Trochlea of humerus
8 years 8 months	Olecranon
9 years 4 months	Lesser troch. femur
9 years 10 months	Pisiform
10 years 4 months	Sesamoids of flex. hall. brevis
10 years 5 months	Hum. lat. epicondyle
10 years 10 months	Tib. tubercle
11 years 0 months	5 metat. prox.
11 years 8 months	Sesamoid of flex. poll. brevis
13 years 3 months	Tubercle, rib 1
13 years 4 months	Ant. inf. iliac spine; Trans. proc. T 1
13 years 5 months	Acromion; iliac crest
13 years 10 months	Coracoid angle
15 years 0 months	Ischial tuber.*
15 years plus	Med. clav.

* Provisional.

FIG. 68.—(Adapted from Francis.)

1. Technique

a) Birth to 5 years (Figs. 64 and 65): Examinations consist of anteroposterior roentgenograms of the left hand and wrist, elbow, shoulder, foot and ankle, knee, and hip.

b) Age 5-15 years (Figs. 67 and 68): Besides the areas mentioned above, additional centers are listed in Figures 67 and 68.

2. Measurements

In compiling standards for the age and sequence of the appearance of ossification centers, Francis, Werle, and Behm used the age when a given center was present in 20% of the number rather than in 50%. Their standards are therefore based on the 80th, and not the 50th, percentile, as is customary. Trial of these standards has confirmed their usefulness as a measure of healthy development.

3. Source of Material

a) Birth to 5 years: The data were derived from roentgenograms of 307 white male and 315 white female normal children from the economically stable classes in Cleveland, Ohio. Each child was examined at 3, 6, 9, and 12 months and thereafter at 6 month intervals to the 5th birthday.

b) Age 5 - 15 years. The same group of children were used with the addition of older siblings and of other preadolescent children from homes of a comparative socioeconomic level. For each age group, 100 children of each sex were selected, allowing a range of not more than 2 weeks on either side of the birthday.

c) Data on ossification and fusion of the sternum (Fig. 66) are obtained from a number of sources and represent a compilation of accumulated information.

*Francis, C. C.: Am. J. Phys. Anthropol. 27:127, 1940.

D. Method of Greulich-Pyle

MALE

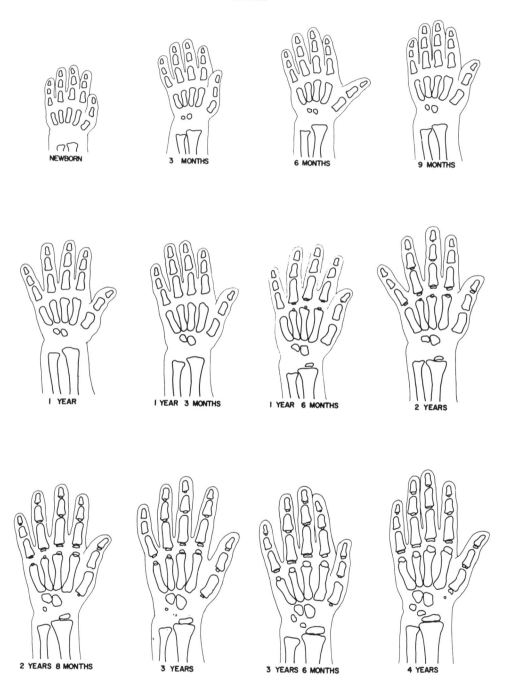

FIG. 69.

Figures 69-73 redrawn from Greulich, W. W., and Pyle, S. I.: *Radiographic Atlas of Skeletal Development of the Hand and Wrist* (2d ed.; Stanford, Calif.: Stanford University Press, 1959).

D. Method of Greulich-Pyle

MALE (continued)

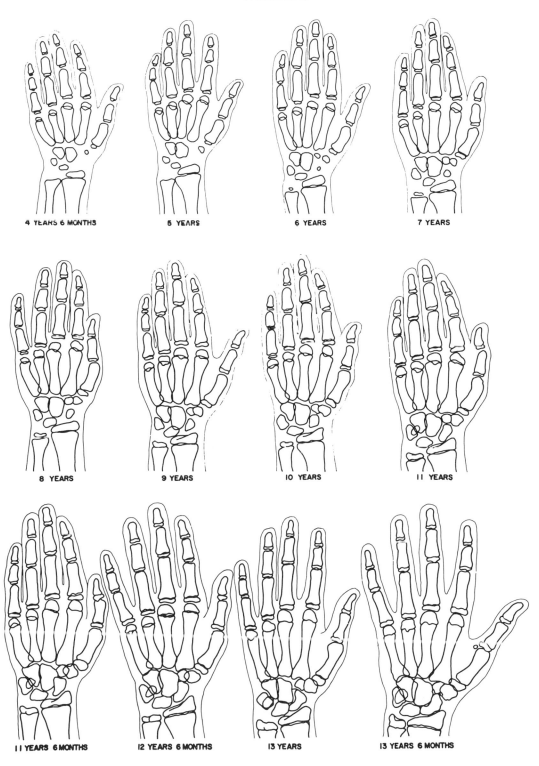

FIG. 70.

D. Method of Greulich-Pyle

MALE (continued)

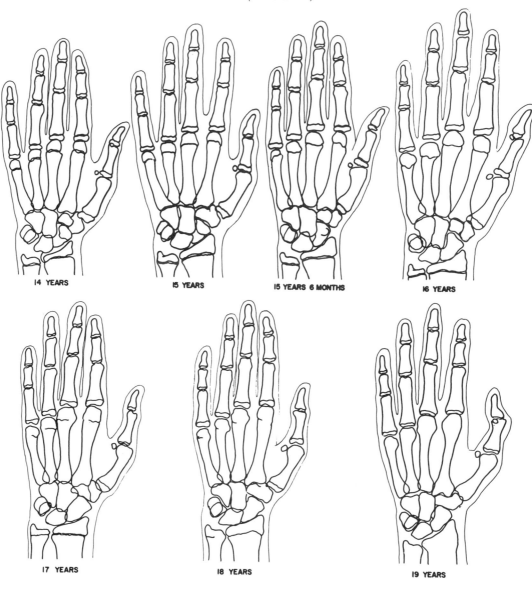

FEMALE

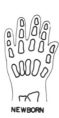
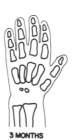
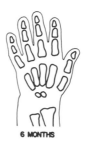
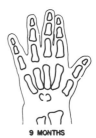

FIG. 71.

D. Method of Greulich-Pyle

FEMALE

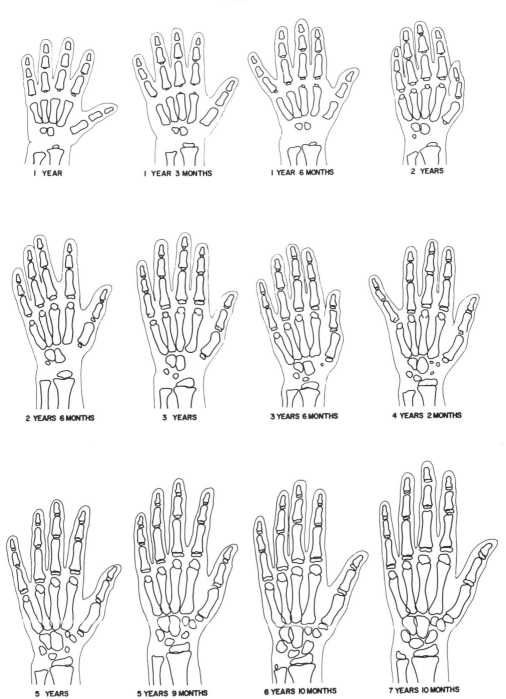

FIG. 72.

D. Method of Greulich-Pyle

FEMALE (continued)

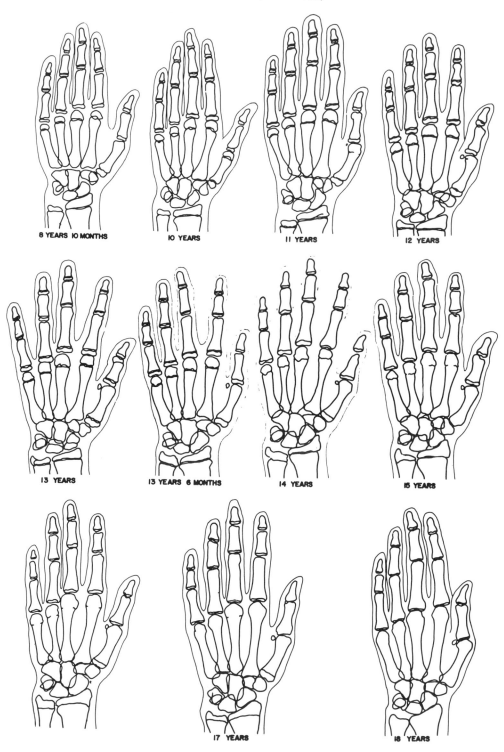

FIG. 73.

D. Method of Greulich-Pyle

1. Technique

   a) Central ray: Perpendicular to plane of film and centered halfway between tips of fingers and distal end of radius.

   b) Position: Posteroanterior.

   c) Target-film distance. Immaterial.

2. Measurements

See Figures 69-73.

The patient's film is compared with the standard of the same sex and nearest chronologic age. It is next compared with adjacent standards, both older and younger than the one which is of the next chronologic age. Select, for a more detailed comparison, the standard which superficially appears to resemble it most closely.

3. Source of Material

Each of the standards was selected from 100 films of children of the same sex and age. The film chosen was selected as the most representative of the central tendency of the group. All children were white; all were born in the United States; and almost all were of North European ancestry. The entire group included 1,000 children.

Note:

Pyle, Waterhouse and Greulich[*] have published a new radiographic reference standard for the assessment of skeletal age from hand-wrist films of children and youths. The reference standard is based in part on the 1959 Greulich and Pyle Atlas which contains one series of reference films for males and another series for females. The new reference standard uses a single series of reference films. The osseous features indicating one and the same skeletal maturity level of each hand-wrist bone appear in the male and female at different chronologic ages. The films in the single film series are calibrated to show the natural chronologic differences between their appearance in males and females.

---

[*]Pyle, S. I., Waterhouse, A. M., and Greulich, W. W.: *A Radiographic Standard of Reference for the Growing Hand and Wrist* (Cleveland, Ohio: The Press of Case Western Reserve University, 1971).

LINEAR GROWTH OF LONG BONES OF EXTREMITIES FROM INFANCY THROUGH ADOLESCENCE*

BOYS – SMOOTHED PERCENTILES AND OBSERVED RANGE FOR ROENTGENOGRAPHIC BONE LENGTHS (CM.)†

A. Arm Bones

Measurements between Epiphysial Plates

Age Yr.–Mo.	Humerus 10%	25%	50%	75%	90%	Range	Radius 10%	25%	50%	75%	90%	Range	Ulna 10%	25%	50%	75%	90%	Range
0–2	6.68	7.02	7.28	7.47	7.65	6.3– 7.9	5.54	5.68	5.85	6.16	6.30	5.4– 6.4	6.29	6.48	6.66	6.89	7.04	6.1– 7.2
0–4	7.43	7.78	8.05	8.29	8.52	7.3– 9.0	6.14	6.29	6.52	6.70	6.95	6.1– 7.0	6.82	7.04	7.22	7.42	7.61	6.8– 7.8
0–6	8.13	8.50	8.80	9.06	9.33	7.8– 9.4	6.60	6.76	7.02	7.24	7.51	6.4– 7.9	7.31	7.55	7.71	7.95	8.22	7.0– 8.7
1–0	9.91	10.25	10.48	10.77	11.20	9.4–11.6	7.68	7.86	8.17	8.42	8.73	7.6– 9.3	8.63	8.85	9.08	9.35	9.69	8.5–10.3
1–6	11.25	11.58	11.84	12.12	12.58	11.0–12.8	8.53	8.78	9.06	9.34	9.67	8.4–10.2	9.55	9.80	10.06	10.37	10.69	9.4–11.4
2–0	12.29	12.72	12.97	13.26	13.71	12.1–14.1	9.23	9.45	9.80	10.10	10.44	9.0–10.2	10.35	10.62	10.90	11.22	11.55	10.1–12.3
2–6	13.12	13.56	13.84	14.13	14.58	12.9–15.0	9.90	10.13	10.47	10.76	11.12	9.6–11.8	11.05	11.33	11.63	11.96	12.29	10.6–13.0
3–0	13.92	14.42	14.65	14.96	15.41	13.6–16.1	10.55	10.78	11.09	11.38	11.75	10.1–12.4	11.70	11.99	12.30	12.64	12.98	11.2–13.6
3–6	14.68	15.21	15.44	15.75	16.21	14.3–16.9	11.13	11.38	11.69	11.97	12.35	10.7–13.0	12.30	12.60	12.93	13.27	13.65	11.8–14.2
4–0	15.41	15.97	16.21	16.52	17.00	15.0–18.0	11.68	11.96	12.26	12.54	12.94	11.1–13.8	12.88	13.19	13.54	13.88	14.30	12.2–15.1
4–6	16.12	16.70	16.95	17.28	17.79	15.8–18.5	12.21	12.51	12.80	13.09	13.51	11.6–14.2	13.44	13.76	14.13	14.48	14.92	12.8–15.5
5–0	16.80	17.39	17.66	18.03	18.57	16.1–19.4	12.73	13.04	13.32	13.61	14.06	11.9–15.0	13.98	14.32	14.70	15.06	15.52	13.1–16.4
5–6	17.47	18.07	18.35	18.76	19.32	17.3–20.3	13.23	13.55	13.82	14.12	14.59	12.8–15.5	14.50	14.86	15.25	15.62	16.08	14.1–17.0
6–0	18.14	18.73	19.03	19.47	20.05	17.4–21.2	13.72	14.01	14.32	14.63	15.12	13.3–16.1	15.00	15.38	15.77	16.15	16.63	14.9–17.6
6–6	18.81	19.38	19.69	20.17	20.76	18.6–22.0	14.19	14.47	14.79	15.13	15.65	13.8–16.8	15.48	15.87	16.27	16.66	17.17	15.2–18.2
7–0	19.46	20.00	20.34	20.86	21.44	19.0–22.9	14.64	14.93	15.26	15.63	16.18	14.1–17.4	15.95	16.35	16.76	17.16	17.71	15.6–18.9
7–6	20.06	20.61	20.97	21.53	22.10	19.6–23.6	15.08	15.38	15.72	16.12	16.69	14.5–18.0	16.41	16.81	17.24	17.66	18.24	16.0–19.5
8–0	20.64	21.19	21.59	22.19	22.75	19.9–24.6	15.50	15.82	16.18	16.60	17.19	14.9–18.6	16.86	17.26	17.70	18.15	18.76	16.3–20.1
8–6	21.19	21.74	22.21	22.83	23.40	20.6–24.6	15.91	16.25	16.63	17.08	17.70	15.5–18.0	17.29	17.71	18.15	18.64	19.28	17.0–19.5
9–0	21.74	22.28	22.81	23.45	24.05	21.2–25.7	16.32	16.68	17.08	17.56	18.21	16.1–20.0	17.72	18.15	18.60	19.13	19.80	17.5–21.2
9–6	22.29	22.82	23.40	24.06	24.69	21.8–26.5	16.72	17.10	17.53	18.04	18.72	16.1–20.0	18.14	18.59	19.05	19.62	20.32	17.8–21.7
10–0	22.79	23.37	23.98	24.67	25.33	22.0–26.9	17.11	17.50	17.97	18.52	19.20	16.9–20.4	18.56	19.03	19.50	20.10	20.84	18.3–22.1
10–6	23.30	23.91	24.56	25.27	25.96	22.6–27.4	17.50	17.90	18.39	18.97	19.68	17.1–20.9	18.97	19.47	19.95	20.58	21.35	18.6–22.5
11–0	23.79	24.44	25.13	25.87	26.59	23.4–28.1	17.88	18.30	18.79	19.40	20.18	17.5–21.4	19.38	19.90	20.39	21.06	21.85	19.3–23.0
11–6	24.27	24.97	25.70	26.48	27.22	22.4–28.5	18.25	18.69	19.19	19.83	20.67	17.8–21.8	19.79	20.31	20.83	21.54	22.35	19.3–23.0
12–0	24.74	25.49	26.28	27.09	27.84	22.8–29.5	18.60	19.07	19.60	20.26	21.15	18.2–22.2	20.20	20.72	21.26	22.01	22.85	19.8–24.0

Measurements Include Epiphyses

Age Yr.–Mo.	Humerus 10%	25%	50%	75%	90%	Range	Radius 10%	25%	50%	75%	90%	Range	Ulna 10%	25%	50%	75%	90%	Range
10–0	24.67	25.31	25.87	26.83	27.58	23.6–29.2	18.42	18.90	19.28	19.85	20.60	18.0–22.2	19.26	19.72	20.27	20.89	21.67	18.9–23.2
10–6	25.12	25.78	26.40	27.37	28.13	24.3–29.8	18.85	19.30	19.71	20.32	21.10	18.4–22.7	19.74	20.21	20.78	21.44	22.27	19.1–23.8
11–0	25.59	26.29	26.98	27.98	28.78	25.0–30.7	19.28	19.71	20.14	20.84	21.63	18.9–23.1	20.23	20.71	21.31	22.01	22.89	19.5–24.4
11–6	26.09	26.83	27.60	28.63	29.48	24.0–31.0	19.73	20.13	20.60	21.39	22.23	19.0–23.7	20.74	21.23	21.86	22.62	23.55	20.8–24.8
12–0	26.62	27.40	28.26	29.33	30.23	24.2–33.3	20.18	20.60	21.11	21.97	22.86	19.4–24.5	21.26	21.76	22.43	23.29	24.32	20.5–26.6
12–6	27.20	28.00	28.98	30.08	31.03	26.8–33.7	20.66	21.09	21.66	22.58	23.53	20.1–25.1	21.81	22.32	23.05	23.99	25.15	20.6–26.9
13–0	27.88	28.70	29.75	30.88	31.88	27.5–34.0	21.16	21.63	22.26	23.23	24.23	20.5–25.0	22.38	22.94	23.71	24.76	25.93	21.6–26.4
13–6	28.69	29.53	30.58	31.75	32.80	27.6–35.1	21.68	22.22	22.96	23.96	24.98	20.7–25.6	22.98	23.63	24.43	25.56	26.68	22.5–27.4
14–0	29.55	30.47	31.48	32.70	33.80	28.5–36.1	22.23	22.90	23.74	24.77	25.80	21.2–26.3	23.62	24.34	25.18	26.33	27.40	22.8–28.2
14–6	30.45	31.43	32.42	33.62	34.59	28.9–36.6	22.85	23.63	24.45	25.39	26.47	21.7–27.1	24.30	25.07	25.94	27.05	28.09	23.5–29.0
15–0	31.40	32.30	33.20	34.38	35.30	30.0–36.6	23.53	24.30	25.13	25.93	27.03	23.4–27.5	25.05	25.82	26.64	27.65	28.72	24.8–29.6
15–6	32.00	32.87	33.87	34.95	35.93	31.0–36.7	24.14	24.84	25.62	26.35	27.46	23.5–27.8	25.68	26.45	27.18	28.10	29.18	25.8–29.8
16–0	32.40	33.33	34.42	35.45	36.82	31.7–37.2	24.52	25.20	25.97	26.66	27.78	23.5–28.4	26.08	26.80	27.57	28.45	29.54	25.3–29.9
16–6	32.72	33.65	34.79	35.84	36.82	29.8–37.8	24.79	25.45	26.20	26.90	27.99	24.5–28.9	26.36	27.05	27.87	28.68	29.82	26.0–30.6
17–0	32.92	33.87	35.02	36.12	37.10	30.4–38.3	24.95	25.59	26.32	27.05	28.14	24.5–29.6	26.50	27.22	28.05	28.85	30.01	26.0–31.1
17–6	33.07	34.04	35.16	36.33	37.28	30.4–38.3	25.00	25.64	26.38	27.14	28.25	24.5–29.6	26.55	27.30	28.14	28.95	30.12	26.0–31.1
18–0	33.17	34.15	35.28	36.46	37.42	31.2–38.7	25.02	25.66	26.42	27.20	28.32	24.5–30.1	26.58	27.34	28.20	29.00	30.17	26.0–31.6

FIG. 74.—(From Maresh, Table 1.)

† Values obtained from about 1600 roentgenograms of the left arm and leg on boys of the Child Research Council study group.

*Maresh, M. M.: A.M.A. J. Dis. Child. 89:725, 1955.

B. Leg Bones

Age Yr.–Mo.	Femur 10%	25%	50%	75%	90%	Range	Tibia 10%	25%	50%	75%	90%	Range	Fibula 10%	25%	50%	75%	90%	Range
Measurements between Epiphyseal Plates																		
0–2	7.76	8.18	8.58	8.85	9.20	7.2– 9.6	6.28	6.65	6.90	7.25	7.67	6.0– 8.3	5.94	6.36	6.65	7.04	7.44	5.6– 8.0
0–4	9.16	9.60	10.00	10.25	10.55	8.8–10.9	7.46	7.75	7.98	8.32	8.73	7.1– 8.8	7.16	7.46	7.70	8.00	8.33	6.8– 8.6
0–6	10.45	10.87	11.21	11.46	11.72	10.2–12.3	8.44	8.70	8.91	9.22	9.63	8.1–10.1	8.03	8.30	8.54	8.84	9.13	7.8– 9.8
1–0	12.75	13.19	13.56	13.96	14.28	12.8–14.9	10.32	10.63	10.87	11.20	11.62	9.9–12.2	9.90	10.21	10.57	10.92	11.26	9.6–11.7
1–6	14.62	15.08	15.50	15.92	16.30	14.5–16.8	11.92	12.26	12.55	12.90	13.34	11.5–13.7	11.48	11.84	12.24	12.61	13.04	11.3–13.5
2–0	16.24	16.73	17.17	17.61	18.03	15.8–18.5	13.22	13.60	13.97	14.35	14.82	13.0–15.1	12.86	13.24	13.68	14.08	14.55	12.7–15.1
2–6	17.66	18.21	18.67	19.13	19.62	16.9–20.0	14.37	14.80	15.22	15.61	16.12	14.0–16.5	14.09	14.50	14.97	15.39	15.88	13.8–16.4
3–0	18.93	19.52	20.00	20.50	21.05	18.2–21.3	15.43	15.87	16.32	16.73	17.26	14.8–17.6	15.22	15.66	16.14	16.58	17.07	14.8–17.6
3–6	20.09	20.70	21.20	21.75	22.35	19.2–22.8	16.43	16.88	17.35	17.78	18.32	16.1–18.9	16.26	16.71	17.20	17.64	18.14	15.9–18.7
4–0	21.23	21.85	22.36	22.97	23.64	19.9–24.8	17.37	17.84	18.33	18.78	19.34	16.8–20.9	17.18	17.65	18.15	18.62	19.15	16.5–20.9
4–6	22.34	22.98	23.51	24.16	24.92	21.0–25.3	18.28	18.77	19.28	19.74	20.31	17.6–21.0	18.08	18.57	19.08	19.52	20.12	17.4–20.7
5–0	23.44	24.10	24.65	25.34	26.18	21.9–27.6	19.15	19.65	20.18	20.66	21.25	18.2–23.0	18.96	19.46	19.98	20.52	21.08	17.9–23.0
5–6	24.52	25.20	25.77	26.51	27.42	23.9–28.3	19.99	20.51	21.06	21.57	22.18	19.6–24.2	19.80	20.31	20.84	21.44	22.03	19.6–24.0
6–0	25.58	26.27	26.87	27.66	28.62	24.7–29.6	20.79	21.34	21.92	22.46	23.10	20.4–25.0	20.62	21.14	21.68	22.33	22.96	20.4–25.0
6–6	26.62	27.33	27.96	28.79	29.78	26.0–30.7	21.57	22.14	22.75	23.35	24.01	21.1–26.4	21.42	21.95	22.50	23.21	23.87	21.0–26.1
7–0	27.64	28.37	29.05	29.90	30.92	26.9–32.9	22.33	22.94	23.57	24.23	24.91	21.6–27.5	22.19	22.74	23.30	24.07	24.77	21.4–27.3
7–6	28.62	29.37	30.06	30.98	32.03	28.2–33.5	23.08	23.73	24.39	25.10	25.81	22.0–28.6	22.94	23.52	24.09	24.92	25.67	22.0–28.4
8–0	29.58	30.35	31.09	32.02	33.10	29.4–35.1	23.83	24.52	25.20	25.96	26.71	23.0–29.6	23.67	24.28	24.87	25.75	26.56	22.8–29.3
8–6	30.52	31.31	32.06	33.03	34.14	30.4–34.6	24.57	25.30	26.01	26.82	27.61	24.1–28.1	24.38	25.02	25.63	26.57	27.44	23.9–28.1
9–0	31.42	32.23	33.02	34.02	35.15	31.3–37.3	25.31	26.05	26.80	27.67	28.50	24.6–31.6	25.07	25.74	26.38	27.37	28.32	24.6–31.0
9–6	32.30	33.13	33.95	35.00	36.14	31.5–38.5	26.03	26.78	27.59	28.50	29.38	24.6–32.5	25.74	26.44	27.12	28.17	29.15	24.8–31.9
10–0	33.16	33.99	34.88	35.96	37.11	33.1–39.2	26.74	27.51	28.37	29.31	30.26	26.2–33.3	26.38	27.13	27.86	28.96	30.06	26.0–32.5
10–6	34.00	34.85	35.78	36.91	38.07	33.3–40.2	27.45	28.23	29.14	30.10	31.13	26.0–34.0	27.01	27.82	28.59	29.75	30.92	26.2–33.3
11–0	34.84	35.70	36.66	37.85	39.03	34.6–41.0	28.15	28.95	29.90	30.89	32.00	27.6–35.2	27.64	28.51	29.31	30.53	31.77	27.1–34.2
11–6	35.67	36.55	37.51	38.79	39.98	33.0–42.0	28.84	29.66	30.66	31.67	32.85	27.0–35.0	28.27	29.19	30.02	31.30	32.61	27.1–35.0
12–0	36.50	37.40	38.41	39.73	40.93	33.7–43.3	29.52	30.37	31.42	32.45	33.70	28.4–36.4	28.90	29.86	30.73	32.06	33.44	27.9–35.3
Measurements Include Epiphyses																		
10–0	37.10	37.70	38.52	39.72	40.95	36.3–43.8	30.28	31.05	32.10	33.11	34.35	29.2–37.9	29.42	30.15	31.05	32.22	33.66	28.8–35.9
10–6	37.85	38.58	39.41	40.67	41.94	36.9–45.3	30.95	31.80	32.92	34.01	35.33	29.6–38.6	30.02	30.80	31.68	32.90	34.36	29.0–36.7
11–0	38.64	39.46	40.39	41.67	43.00	38.0–45.7	31.70	32.59	33.80	34.96	36.34	30.8–39.8	30.65	31.50	32.44	33.68	35.16	30.2–37.6
11–6	39.46	40.35	41.37	42.70	44.10	36.5–46.8	32.50	33.45	34.72	35.96	37.37	31.0–40.6	31.34	32.26	33.27	34.53	36.03	30.7–38.7
12–0	40.32	41.26	42.40	43.80	45.26	37.2–48.0	33.35	34.38	35.70	36.99	38.42	32.2–41.3	32.08	33.06	34.16	35.44	36.97	30.7–38.9
12–6	41.22	42.19	43.41	44.95	46.45	40.7–48.8	34.27	35.35	36.73	38.04	39.50	33.2–42.3	32.87	33.91	35.10	36.43	38.00	32.1–39.7
13–0	42.15	43.15	44.50	46.18	47.67	41.0–49.3	35.25	36.38	37.80	39.13	40.64	34.2–42.7	33.73	34.83	36.10	37.51	39.15	33.0–40.7
13–6	43.12	44.18	45.60	47.45	48.97	40.5–50.9	36.36	37.57	39.00	40.40	41.93	34.5–43.5	34.64	35.81	37.25	38.72	40.43	33.1–41.2
14–0	44.10	45.27	46.77	48.70	50.22	41.3–51.9	37.55	38.70	39.95	41.37	43.03	36.8–44.5	35.70	36.89	38.25	39.79	41.57	35.1–42.6
14–6	45.18	46.43	47.96	49.80	51.36	41.6–52.5	38.53	39.57	40.80	42.25	43.95	35.9–45.2	36.70	37.89	39.15	40.74	42.57	34.8–43.1
15–0	46.30	47.60	49.00	50.65	52.23	44.8–53.7	39.17	40.25	41.50	42.98	44.72	38.5–45.9	37.55	38.65	39.94	41.56	43.43	36.6–44.2
15–6	47.25	48.45	49.80	51.32	52.90	46.4–54.2	39.61	40.75	42.10	43.62	45.39	37.9–47.0	38.08	39.20	40.54	42.20	44.11	37.0–45.6
16–0	47.67	48.83	50.21	51.82	53.38	45.3–54.9	39.82	41.07	42.50	44.05	45.90	38.6–48.2	38.36	39.50	40.95	42.66	44.63	36.7–46.3
16–6	47.95	49.07	50.40	52.15	53.75	47.1–56.5	39.95	41.20	42.75	44.33	46.21	39.4–48.7	38.43	39.62	41.22	42.99	45.03	38.2–46.3
17–0	48.10	49.14	50.45	52.38	54.02	47.0–57.0	40.04	41.27	42.90	44.51	46.42	39.1–49.1	38.47	39.66	41.37	43.22	45.33	37.9–46.8
17–6	48.17	49.19	50.48	52.52	54.20	47.0–57.0	40.08	41.30	42.98	44.60	46.51	39.1–49.1	38.49	39.69	41.46	43.36	45.54	37.9–46.8
18–0	48.20	49.22	50.50	52.60	54.30	48.1–57.4	40.10	41.33	43.03	44.66	46.60	39.0–49.6	38.50	39.70	41.50	43.45	45.68	37.9–47.5

FIG. 74 (Cont.)

GIRLS — SMOOTHED PERCENTILES AND OBSERVED RANGE FOR ROENTGENOGRAPHIC BONE LENGTHS (CM.)[†]

A. Arm Bones

Measurements between Epiphysial Plates

Age Yr.–Mo.	Humerus 10%	25%	50%	75%	90%	Range	Radius 10%	25%	50%	75%	90%	Range	Ulna 10%	25%	50%	75%	90%	Range
0-2	6.72	6.91	7.12	7.30	7.50	6.0-7.7	5.43	5.58	5.72	5.88	6.05	5.2-6.5	6.08	6.30	6.50	6.65	6.82	5.8-7.2
0-4	7.52	7.73	8.00	8.17	8.38	7.4-8.8	5.93	6.11	6.28	6.46	6.64	5.7-7.0	6.59	6.84	7.05	7.21	7.38	6.4-7.9
0-6	8.22	8.44	8.74	8.89	9.12	7.7-9.5	6.37	6.51	6.74	6.95	7.14	6.0-7.5	7.09	7.35	7.58	7.75	7.92	6.7-8.2
1-0	9.77	10.04	10.38	10.60	10.86	8.8-11.4	7.42	7.64	7.85	8.10	8.31	7.1-8.6	8.27	8.56	8.82	9.06	9.32	7.9-9.7
1-6	11.02	11.32	11.70	11.98	12.27	10.6-12.7	8.22	8.48	8.74	9.00	9.24	7.9-9.7	9.24	9.55	9.84	10.11	10.41	8.8-10.9
2-0	12.07	12.40	12.80	13.10	13.42	11.5-14.0	8.92	9.20	9.50	9.77	10.04	8.5-10.4	10.00	10.34	10.66	10.95	11.27	9.3-11.6
2-6	12.94	13.32	13.75	14.09	14.44	12.6-14.9	9.55	9.85	10.18	10.47	10.75	8.7-11.1	10.69	11.05	11.39	11.70	12.04	9.8-12.4
3-0	13.73	14.13	14.58	14.99	15.39	13.2-15.7	10.12	10.45	10.80	11.12	11.41	9.9-11.8	11.32	11.70	12.07	12.39	12.75	11.0-13.2
3-6	14.49	14.91	15.38	15.84	16.28	13.8-16.7	10.66	11.01	11.39	11.73	12.05	10.3-12.5	11.90	12.31	12.71	13.04	13.42	11.6-13.9
4-0	15.21	15.66	16.15	16.66	17.14	14.3-17.4	11.18	11.55	11.95	12.33	12.68	10.8-12.9	12.45	12.88	13.32	13.67	14.06	12.1-14.4
4-6	15.90	16.37	16.89	17.44	17.97	15.0-18.5	11.68	12.06	12.48	12.91	13.30	11.3-13.8	12.98	13.43	13.90	14.29	14.69	12.6-15.2
5-0	16.56	17.05	17.60	18.21	18.77	15.8-19.5	12.16	12.55	12.99	13.47	13.90	11.8-15.0	13.49	13.96	14.45	14.89	15.30	13.1-16.5
5-6	17.19	17.71	18.29	18.94	19.54	16.1-20.1	12.62	13.02	13.48	14.01	14.48	12.3-15.4	13.99	14.47	14.98	15.46	15.90	13.5-16.5
6-0	17.80	18.35	18.95	19.64	20.29	16.8-20.7	13.06	13.49	13.97	14.53	15.03	12.7-16.5	14.47	14.96	15.50	16.02	16.48	14.0-17.0
6-6	18.40	18.98	19.60	20.32	21.01	17.4-22.2	13.49	13.95	14.45	15.05	15.55	13.1-17.2	14.94	15.45	16.01	16.56	17.05	14.6-18.4
7-0	18.99	19.60	20.25	20.99	21.71	18.2-23.3	13.91	14.41	14.92	15.56	16.06	13.6-17.2	15.41	15.94	16.51	17.09	17.60	15.0-19.1
7-6	19.56	20.21	20.89	21.65	22.40	18.6-23.1	14.33	14.86	15.39	16.05	16.56	14.0-18.1	15.87	16.42	17.01	17.62	18.13	15.5-18.6
8-0	20.12	20.82	21.51	22.30	23.07	19.4-24.4	14.74	15.29	15.86	16.53	17.04	14.5-18.1	16.32	16.90	17.50	18.14	18.65	15.9-20.1
8-6	20.66	21.42	22.13	22.94	23.73	19.8-24.4	15.15	15.71	16.33	17.00	17.51	14.9-18.5	16.77	17.38	17.99	18.66	19.16	16.4-19.6
9-0	21.19	22.01	22.75	23.58	24.40	20.8-25.1	15.55	16.13	16.80	17.47	18.00	15.6-19.7	17.20	17.85	18.47	19.18	19.68	16.8-20.4
9-6	21.71	22.59	23.38	24.24	25.08	20.8-26.5	15.96	16.54	17.26	17.96	18.50	16.0-21.4	17.62	18.30	18.94	19.70	20.22	17.2-21.7
10-0	22.23	23.17	24.03	24.91	25.78	21.4-26.4	16.38	16.97	17.72	18.45	19.02	16.4-21.4	18.04	18.73	19.44	20.23	20.79	17.7-21.5
10-6	22.77	23.76	24.70	25.60	26.51	21.7-28.2	16.81	17.42	18.20	18.95	19.55	16.7-21.1	18.50	19.20	19.99	20.78	21.40	18.0-23.8
11-0	23.32	24.36	25.38	26.31	27.25	22.0-28.0	17.25	17.89	18.70	19.48	20.13	17.0-21.9	18.97	19.69	20.57	21.37	22.03	18.5-23.6
11-6	23.88	24.98	26.07	27.03	28.01	22.4-29.5	17.72	18.39	19.23	20.03	20.77	17.2-21.9	19.46	20.24	21.17	21.98	22.68	19.1-24.5
12-0	24.45	25.62	26.78	27.76	28.78	22.8-30.0	18.22	18.93	19.80	20.63	21.44	17.5-22.3	19.98	20.82	21.80	22.60	23.33	19.6-25.1

Measurements Include Epiphyses

Age Yr.–Mo.	Humerus 10%	25%	50%	75%	90%	Range	Radius 10%	25%	50%	75%	90%	Range	Ulna 10%	25%	50%	75%	90%	Range
10-0	23.80	24.66	25.80	26.73	27.50	23.0-28.2	17.50	18.32	19.03	19.87	20.62	17.0-21.0	18.95	19.75	20.50	21.40	22.20	18.6-22.9
10-6	24.55	25.52	26.73	27.73	28.66	23.6-30.7	17.94	18.85	19.65	20.61	21.39	17.5-23.0	19.53	20.36	21.28	22.20	23.07	19.0-25.1
11-0	25.28	26.31	27.60	28.64	29.68	23.8-30.9	18.41	19.38	20.28	21.33	22.12	17.8-23.0	20.12	20.97	22.00	22.94	23.83	19.7-24.6
11-6	25.98	27.06	28.38	29.46	30.60	24.2-32.0	18.93	19.92	20.90	21.99	22.78	18.2-23.7	20.70	21.58	22.65	23.60	24.51	20.2-25.4
12-0	26.65	27.75	29.09	30.19	31.43	24.8-32.9	19.45	20.48	21.50	22.59	23.39	18.8-24.5	21.28	22.18	23.24	24.20	25.12	20.5-26.8
12-6	27.28	28.38	29.72	30.86	32.18	25.4-33.2	19.97	21.06	22.07	23.10	23.89	19.3-24.8	21.85	22.77	23.75	24.70	25.62	21.0-26.9
13-0	27.87	28.97	30.30	31.46	32.85	26.1-33.8	20.49	21.57	22.55	23.54	24.29	19.9-24.8	22.40	23.28	24.18	25.13	26.04	21.5-27.2
13-6	28.42	29.51	30.82	32.00	33.40	26.6-34.5	21.00	22.03	22.98	23.89	24.60	20.5-24.9	22.92	23.73	24.57	25.48	26.40	22.1-27.2
14-0	28.92	30.00	31.30	32.40	33.77	27.7-35.2	21.50	22.45	23.34	24.12	24.80	20.9-25.4	23.36	24.13	24.89	25.76	26.69	22.6-27.2
14-6	29.37	30.42	31.70	32.66	33.95	28.0-35.9	21.88	22.80	23.62	24.28	24.94	21.4-25.9	23.69	24.47	25.16	25.92	26.90	22.9-27.5
15-0	29.72	30.74	32.00	32.79	34.06	28.5-36.1	22.13	23.02	23.82	24.38	25.03	21.6-26.1	23.95	24.76	25.37	26.04	27.03	23.0-27.7
15-6	29.92	30.92	32.15	32.88	34.10	28.8-36.5	22.22	23.12	23.92	24.45	25.08	21.8-26.2	24.12	24.98	25.51	26.14	27.12	23.4-28.1
16-0	30.02	31.01	32.20	32.92	34.10	28.8-36.5	22.25	23.15	23.98	24.48	25.10	21.8-26.2	24.22	25.10	25.60	26.21	27.16	23.4-28.1

FIG. 75.—(From Maresh, Table 2.)

† Values obtained from over 1600 roentgenograms of the left arm and leg on girls of the Child Research Council study group.

LINEAR GROWTH OF LONG BONES OF EXTREMITIES FROM INFANCY THROUGH ADOLESCENCE

B. Leg Bones

Age Yr.–Mo.	Femur						Tibia						Fibula					
	10%	25%	50%	75%	90%	Range	10%	25%	50%	75%	90%	Range	10%	25%	50%	75%	90%	Range
							Measurements between Epiphysial Plates											
0–2	8.20	8.50	8.72	9.00	9.28	7.8- 9.7	6.32	6.67	7.00	7.28	7.58	6.0- 8.0	6.06	6.30	6.55	6.86	7.16	5.7- 7.5
0–4	9.43	9.78	10.00	10.25	10.50	9.4-10.9	7.35	7.69	8.03	8.30	8.60	7.0- 8.8	7.02	7.36	7.67	7.90	8.21	6.7- 8.4
0–6	10.57	10.91	11.15	11.36	11.58	9.8-12.0	8.20	8.60	8.87	9.17	9.48	7.3- 9.8	7.74	8.16	8.52	8.78	9.00	6.9- 9.4
1–0	12.67	13.06	13.36	13.80	14.18	12.3-14.8	10.12	10.50	10.77	11.10	11.51	9.6-12.0	9.57	10.13	10.52	10.86	11.15	9.3-11.6
1–6	14.44	14.88	15.26	15.80	16.30	14.2-16.7	11.64	12.05	12.37	12.75	13.20	11.2-13.5	11.23	11.73	12.17	12.56	12.90	10.6-13.4
2–0	16.00	16.47	16.89	17.48	18.02	15.8-18.7	12.92	13.39	13.75	14.14	14.65	12.4-15.2	12.55	13.08	13.54	13.96	14.36	12.0-15.1
2–6	17.39	17.89	18.37	19.00	19.58	17.0-20.1	14.03	14.54	15.00	15.42	15.95	13.7-16.4	13.74	14.29	14.78	15.22	15.67	13.3-16.3
3–0	18.64	19.19	19.74	20.40	21.02	17.8-21.4	14.99	15.52	16.10	16.57	17.15	14.0-17.8	14.82	15.40	15.93	16.40	16.88	14.1-17.7
3–6	19.80	20.39	21.01	21.73	22.41	19.1-22.9	15.87	16.52	17.14	17.67	18.30	15.0-19.1	15.83	16.45	17.02	17.51	18.02	15.1-18.8
4–0	20.90	21.54	22.24	23.02	23.76	20.1-24.2	16.71	17.46	18.15	18.73	19.43	15.7-20.0	16.76	17.42	18.03	18.58	19.12	15.8-19.8
4–6	21.96	22.66	23.44	24.27	25.07	21.2-25.8	17.55	18.38	19.12	19.75	20.54	16.7-21.1	17.58	18.30	18.96	19.62	20.20	16.6-21.0
5–0	23.00	23.76	24.63	25.50	26.35	22.4-27.1	18.38	19.28	20.06	20.74	21.62	17.5-22.6	18.35	19.15	19.85	20.62	21.26	17.4-22.4
5–6	24.02	24.84	25.79	26.71	27.60	23.3-28.2	19.20	20.16	20.96	21.71	22.63	18.3-23.5	19.12	19.97	20.73	21.59	22.29	18.3-23.1
6–0	25.02	25.92	26.94	27.89	28.81	24.2-30.0	20.00	21.01	21.83	22.67	23.61	19.3-24.3	19.88	20.78	21.60	22.52	23.27	19.6-24.0
6–6	26.02	26.99	28.07	29.04	29.98	25.2-30.8	20.77	21.84	22.70	23.60	24.57	20.0-25.7	20.64	21.59	22.46	23.41	24.21	20.0-25.3
7–0	27.01	28.06	29.16	30.15	31.10	26.0-32.2	21.54	22.67	23.56	24.51	25.51	20.7-26.7	21.39	22.39	23.32	24.27	25.09	20.6-26.3
7–6	27.99	29.11	30.22	31.22	32.18	26.8-34.0	22.31	23.50	24.41	25.42	26.45	21.5-27.5	22.13	23.19	24.18	25.10	25.91	21.3-27.2
8–0	28.94	30.11	31.25	32.25	33.21	27.8-34.3	23.07	24.32	25.25	26.32	27.38	22.3-28.4	22.87	23.98	25.04	25.91	26.74	22.1-27.9
8–6	29.84	31.06	32.25	33.26	34.24	28.8-34.9	23.80	25.12	26.09	27.22	28.28	23.1-29.2	23.58	24.76	25.88	26.74	27.58	22.7-28.6
9–0	30.69	31.95	33.22	34.24	35.26	29.6-36.2	24.50	25.91	26.93	28.02	29.18	23.7-30.1	24.26	25.52	26.70	27.62	28.52	23.4-29.5
9–6	31.50	32.80	34.14	35.18	36.28	30.5-38.1	25.19	26.67	27.77	29.02	30.10	24.4-31.3	24.92	26.25	27.48	28.60	29.60	24.1-30.7
10–0	32.28	33.62	35.02	36.17	37.30	31.3-38.3	25.87	27.42	28.59	29.98	31.05	25.3-31.9	25.61	26.99	28.28	29.54	30.65	24.8-31.4
10–6	33.03	34.47	35.96	37.20	38.35	32.2-41.6	26.54	28.17	29.40	30.85	32.01	25.9-33.8	26.31	27.77	29.12	30.46	31.67	25.4-33.0
11–0	33.78	35.36	36.95	38.28	39.45	33.2-43.2	27.28	28.95	30.26	31.80	32.98	26.5-35.0	27.02	28.56	29.90	31.31	32.61	25.9-33.9
11–6	34.60	36.29	38.05	39.40	40.60	34.0-44.1	28.10	29.77	31.18	32.77	33.99	27.3-35.8	27.72	29.32	30.60	32.08	33.45	26.7-35.0
12–0	35.50	37.35	39.32	40.55	41.85	35.2-44.9	29.02	30.71	32.18	33.80	35.10	28.1-36.6	28.40	30.02	31.26	32.80	34.30	27.3-35.7
							Measurements Include Epiphyses											
10–0	35.57	37.05	39.03	40.15	41.50	34.6-42.0	29.51	31.10	32.55	34.12	35.22	28.4-35.9	28.47	30.12	31.55	32.70	33.75	27.6-34.6
10–6	36.39	37.93	40.02	41.50	43.15	35.5-46.3	30.34	32.00	33.64	35.30	36.60	29.2-37.8	29.13	30.82	32.28	33.88	35.12	28.3-36.1
11–0	37.32	38.90	41.02	42.72	44.41	36.6-47.8	31.18	32.92	34.64	36.35	37.76	30.3-39.0	29.87	31.58	33.04	34.86	36.12	28.9-37.3
11–6	38.33	40.04	42.08	43.85	45.49	37.5-48.7	32.03	33.86	35.52	37.28	38.70	31.1-40.4	30.68	32.42	33.90	35.74	37.03	29.7-38.4
12–0	39.40	41.21	43.30	44.90	46.48	38.9-49.3	32.91	34.80	36.30	38.13	39.49	32.0-41.0	31.47	33.26	34.75	36.53	37.83	30.4-39.2
12–6	40.34	42.22	44.37	45.83	47.35	39.8-48.4	33.74	35.66	37.00	38.88	40.14	32.7-41.0	32.25	34.06	35.55	37.22	38.56	31.2-39.4
13–0	41.18	43.10	45.27	46.62	48.09	39.8-51.0	34.50	36.39	37.66	39.47	40.67	33.6-42.1	33.01	34.83	36.28	37.80	39.18	32.0-40.6
13–6	41.95	43.90	46.05	47.24	48.67	41.5-49.1	35.21	37.02	38.28	39.93	41.08	34.3-42.8	33.63	35.46	36.87	38.26	39.65	32.6-41.3
14–0	42.65	44.58	46.65	47.69	49.10	41.7-52.1	35.80	37.55	38.78	40.28	41.39	34.6-43.4	34.13	35.94	37.33	38.61	39.98	32.6-41.8
14–6	43.31	45.09	47.05	48.03	49.42	42.3-50.1	36.21	37.92	39.17	40.51	41.58	34.9-43.3	34.51	36.30	37.70	38.86	40.20	33.1-41.8
15–0	43.86	45.41	47.23	48.27	49.58	42.3-52.0	36.50	38.15	39.36	40.66	41.67	34.8-41.9	34.82	36.60	37.94	39.00	40.32	33.5-40.6
15–6	44.17	45.60	47.23	48.37	49.65	42.2-52.0	36.69	38.30	39.45	40.75	41.70	34.8-42.0	35.05	36.83	38.06	39.07	40.36	33.4-40.7
16–0	44.35	45.66	47.23	48.40	49.65	42.2-52.0	36.78	38.37	39.50	40.78	41.70	34.8-42.0	35.20	36.98	38.10	39.10	40.36	33.4-40.7

FIG. 75 (Cont.)

LINEAR GROWTH OF LONG BONES OF EXTREMITIES FROM INFANCY THROUGH ADOLESCENCE

1. *Technique*

    a) Central ray: Perpendicular to plane of film.

    b) Position: Anteroposterior.

    c) Target-film distance: 7½ feet (228.6 cm.) used to reduce distortion to a minimum.

2. *Measurements*

    See Figures 74 and 75.

    No corrections of the measurements have been made for distortion. Calculation of this magnification shows it to be between 1.0 and 1.5% at this target-film distance.

    The lengths of the bones are the greatest possible length of the shaft between the epiphysial plates. In the preadolescent and later years the ossified epiphyses were included and the measurement made from the most proximal edge of the upper epiphysis to the most distal edge of the lower epiphysis. When the lower epiphysis had a visible styloid process, such as the radius or ulna, that length was included in the measurement.

3. *Source of Material*

    Measurements were made on the roentgenograms of about 175 normal subjects, ranging in age from less than 1 year to over 18 years for a few slowly maturing boys. The number of sets of films on each subject ranged from under 10 for infants and young children to over 25 for those who were adolescent or skeletally mature. The subjects are from a selected group of families in the Child Research Council, but it is quite probable that the described patterns of growth are not unique to this group.

    Note:

    Maresh has published* a series of measurements from roentgenograms which include heart size, long-bone length, bone length relative to height, and width measurements in bone, fat and muscle.

---

*Maresh, M. M.: in McCammon, R. W. (ed.): *Human Growth and Development* (Springfield, Ill.: Charles C Thomas, Publisher, 1970), pp. 155-200.

SURGICAL GROWTH ARREST FOR FEMUR AND TIBIA*

Figure 76 may be used in estimating the amounts of growth which may be inhibited in the distal end of the normal femur or proximal end of the normal tibia by epiphysial arrest at the skeletal ages indicated on the base line.

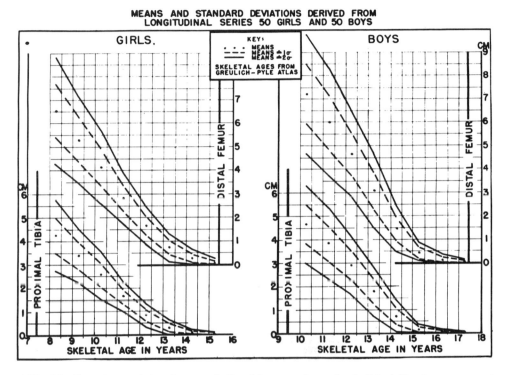

FIG. 76.—Growth remaining in normal distal femur and proximal tibia following consecutive skeletal age levels. (From Anderson, Chart III.)

*Anderson, M., et al.: J. Bone & Joint Surg. 45-A:1, 1963.

SURGICAL GROWTH ARREST FOR FEMUR AND TIBIA

1. Technique

Orthodiograms were made with three separate exposures of the lower extremity. The three exposures were processed on a continuous film up to 44 inches in length.

a) Central ray: Directed successively over hip, knee, and ankle joint.
b) Position: Anteroposterior.
c) Target-film distance: 6 feet.

2. Measurements

In the use of Figure 76, the factors discussed below should be considered. A child who has been consistently tall will grow appreciably more over a number of years than will a child who has always been short. Knowledge of the relative heights of other members of his family is also of some assistance, particularly if there is variation in the family pattern. The chart shows the extent of normal deviation. A child who is showing marked inhibition on the shorter side will obtain proportionately less than the average corrected indicated on the chart. A child whose serial skeletal ages indicate increasingly advanced maturation will likewise grow less than the average amount before maturity. An extremely tall individual, on the other hand, who has normal epiphyses on the shorter extremity might be expected to get a somewhat greater-than-average correction from an epiphysial arrest; and, conversely, less than the average amount may be gained in a very short child. The amount of correction which may be anticipated in a given child after epiphysial arrest may thus be estimated by locating on the growth chart the probable limits of his growth as it will be influenced by his particular problems.

3. Source of Material

Data derived from measurements of normal lower extremities in 50 girls and 50 boys where growth had been recorded at annual intervals over the last 8 years preceding epiphysial fusion.

AVERAGE BOYS — PERCENTAGES AND ESTIMATED MATURE HEIGHTS FOR BOYS WITH SKELETAL AGES WITHIN ONE YEAR OF THEIR CHRONOLOGIC AGES

Skeletal Ages 7 through 12 Years

Skeletal Age Ht. (inches)	7-0	7-3	7-6	7-9	8-0	8-3	8-6	8-9	9-0	9-3	9-6	9-9	10-0	10-3	10-6	10-9	11-0	11-3	11-6	11-9	12-0	12-3	12-6	12-9
% of Mature Height	69.5	70.2	70.9	71.6	72.3	73.1	73.9	74.6	75.2	76.1	76.9	77.7	78.4	79.1	79.5	80.0	80.4	81.2	81.8	82.7	83.4	84.3	85.3	86.3
42	60.4																							
43	61.9	61.3	60.6	60.1																				
44	63.3	62.7	62.1	61.5	60.9	60.2																		
45	64.7	64.1	63.5	62.8	62.2	61.6	60.9	60.3																
46	66.2	65.5	64.9	64.2	63.6	62.9	62.2	61.7	61.2	60.4														
47	67.6	67.0	66.3	65.6	65.0	64.3	63.6	63.0	62.5	61.8	61.1	60.5												
48	69.1	68.4	67.7	67.0	66.4	65.7	65.0	64.3	63.8	63.1	62.4	61.8	61.2	60.7	60.4	60.0								
49	70.5	69.8	69.1	68.4	67.8	67.0	66.3	65.7	65.2	64.4	63.7	63.1	62.5	61.9	61.6	61.3	60.9	60.3						
50	71.9	71.2	70.5	69.8	69.2	68.4	67.7	67.0	66.5	65.7	65.0	64.4	63.8	63.2	62.9	62.5	62.2	61.6	61.1	60.5				
51	73.4	72.6	71.9	71.2	70.5	69.8	69.0	68.4	67.8	67.0	66.3	65.6	65.1	64.5	64.2	63.8	63.4	62.8	62.3	61.7	61.1	60.5	59.8	
52	74.8	74.1	73.3	72.6	71.9	71.1	70.4	69.7	69.1	68.3	67.6	66.9	66.3	65.7	65.4	65.0	64.7	64.0	63.6	62.9	62.3	61.7	61.0	60.3
53	76.3	75.5	74.8	74.0	73.3	72.5	71.7	71.0	70.5	69.6	68.9	68.2	67.6	67.0	66.7	66.3	65.9	65.3	64.8	64.1	63.5	62.9	62.1	61.4
54	77.7	76.9	76.2	75.4	74.7	73.9	73.1	72.4	71.8	71.0	70.2	69.5	68.9	68.3	67.9	67.5	67.2	66.5	66.0	65.3	64.7	64.1	63.3	62.6
55	79.1	78.3	77.6	76.8	76.1	75.2	74.4	73.7	73.1	72.3	71.5	70.8	70.2	69.5	69.2	68.8	68.4	67.7	67.2	66.5	65.9	65.2	64.5	63.7
56	80.6	79.8	79.0	78.2	77.5	76.6	75.8	75.1	74.5	73.6	72.8	72.1	71.4	70.8	70.4	70.0	69.7	69.0	68.5	67.7	67.1	66.4	65.6	64.9
57			80.4	79.6	78.8	78.0	77.1	76.4	75.8	74.9	74.1	73.4	72.7	72.1	71.7	71.3	70.9	70.2	69.7	68.9	68.3	67.6	66.8	66.0
58					80.2	79.3	78.5	77.7	77.1	76.2	75.4	74.6	74.0	73.3	73.0	72.5	72.1	71.4	70.9	70.1	69.5	68.8	68.0	67.2
59						80.7	79.8	79.1	78.5	77.5	76.7	75.9	75.3	74.6	74.2	73.8	73.4	72.7	72.1	71.3	70.7	70.0	69.2	68.4
60							80.4	79.8	78.8	78.0	77.2	76.5	75.9	75.5	75.0	74.6	73.9	73.3	72.6	71.9	71.2	70.3	69.5	
61									80.2	79.3	78.5	77.8	77.1	76.7	76.3	75.9	75.1	74.6	73.8	73.1	72.4	71.5	70.7	
62										80.6	79.8	79.1	78.4	78.0	77.5	77.1	76.4	75.8	75.0	74.3	73.5	72.7	71.8	
63												80.4	79.6	79.2	78.8	78.1	77.6	77.0	76.2	75.5	74.7	73.9	73.0	
64													80.9	80.5	80.0	79.6	78.8	78.2	77.4	76.7	75.9	75.0	74.2	
65																80.8	80.0	79.5	78.6	77.9	77.1	76.2	75.3	
66																		80.7	79.8	79.1	78.3	77.4	76.5	
67																				80.3	79.5	78.5	77.6	
68																					80.7	79.7	78.8	
69																						80.9	80.0	

FIG. 77.

AVERAGE BOYS — PERCENTAGES AND ESTIMATED MATURE HEIGHTS FOR BOYS WITH SKELETAL AGES WITHIN ONE YEAR OF THEIR CHRONOLOGIC AGES

Skeletal Ages 13 Years to Maturity

Skeletal Age Ht. (inches)	13-0	13-3	13-6	13-9	14-0	14-3	14-6	14-9	15-0	15-3	15-6	15-9	16-0	16-3	16-6	16-9	17-0	17-3	17-6	17-9	18-0	18-3	18-6
% of Mature Height	87.6	89.0	90.2	91.4	92.7	93.8	94.8	95.8	96.8	97.3	97.6	98.0	98.2	98.5	98.7	98.9	99.1	99.3	99.4	99.5	99.6	99.8	100.0
53	60.5																						
54	61.6	60.7																					
55	62.8	61.8	61.0	60.2																			
56	63.9	62.9	62.1	61.3	60.4																		
57	65.1	64.0	63.2	62.4	61.5	60.8	60.1																
58	66.2	65.2	64.3	63.5	62.6	61.8	61.2	60.5															
59	67.4	66.3	65.4	64.6	63.6	62.9	62.2	61.6	61.0	60.6	60.5	60.2	60.1										
60	68.5	67.4	66.5	65.6	64.7	64.0	63.3	62.6	62.0	61.7	61.5	61.2	61.1	60.9	60.8	60.7	60.5	60.4	60.4	60.3	60.2	60.1	60.0
61	69.6	68.5	67.6	66.7	65.8	65.0	64.3	63.7	63.0	62.7	62.5	62.2	62.1	61.9	61.8	61.7	61.6	61.4	61.4	61.3	61.2	61.1	61.0
62	70.8	69.7	68.7	67.8	66.9	66.1	65.4	64.7	64.1	63.7	63.5	63.3	63.1	62.9	62.8	62.7	62.6	62.4	62.4	62.3	62.2	62.1	62.0
63	71.9	70.8	69.8	68.9	68.0	67.2	66.5	65.8	65.1	64.7	64.5	64.3	64.2	64.0	63.8	63.7	63.6	63.4	63.4	63.3	63.3	63.1	63.0
64	73.1	71.9	71.0	70.0	69.0	68.2	67.5	66.8	66.1	65.8	65.6	65.3	65.2	65.0	64.8	64.7	64.6	64.4	64.4	64.3	64.3	64.1	64.0
65	74.2	73.0	72.1	71.1	70.1	69.3	68.6	67.8	67.2	66.8	66.6	66.3	66.2	66.0	65.9	65.7	65.6	65.5	65.4	65.3	65.3	65.1	65.0
66	75.3	74.2	73.2	72.2	71.2	70.4	69.6	68.9	68.2	67.8	67.6	67.3	67.2	67.0	66.9	66.7	66.6	66.5	66.4	66.3	66.3	66.1	66.0
67	76.5	75.3	74.3	73.3	72.3	71.4	70.7	69.9	69.2	68.9	68.6	68.4	68.2	68.0	67.9	67.7	67.6	67.5	67.4	67.4	67.3	67.1	67.0
68	77.6	76.4	75.4	74.4	73.4	72.5	71.7	71.0	70.3	69.9	69.7	69.4	69.2	69.0	68.9	68.8	68.6	68.5	68.4	68.3	68.3	68.1	68.0
69	78.8	77.5	76.5	75.5	74.4	73.6	72.8	72.0	71.3	70.9	70.7	70.4	70.3	70.0	69.9	69.8	69.6	69.5	69.4	69.3	69.3	69.1	69.0
70	79.9	78.7	77.6	76.6	75.5	74.6	73.8	73.1	72.3	71.9	71.7	71.4	71.3	71.1	70.9	70.8	70.6	70.5	70.4	70.4	70.3	70.1	70.0
71		79.8	78.7	77.7	76.6	75.7	74.9	74.1	73.4	73.0	72.7	72.4	72.3	72.1	71.9	71.8	71.6	71.5	71.4	71.4	71.3	71.1	71.0
72		80.9	79.8	78.8	77.7	76.8	75.9	75.2	74.4	74.0	73.8	73.5	73.3	73.1	73.0	72.8	72.7	72.5	72.4	72.4	72.3	72.1	72.0
73			80.9	79.9	78.7	77.8	77.0	76.2	75.4	75.0	74.8	74.5	74.3	74.1	74.0	73.8	73.7	73.5	73.4	73.4	73.3	73.1	73.0
74				79.8	78.9	78.1	77.2	76.4	76.0	75.8	75.5	75.4	75.1	75.0	74.8	74.7	74.5	74.4	74.4	74.3	74.1	74.0	
75				80.9	80.0	79.1	78.8	77.3	77.1	76.8	76.5	76.4	76.1	76.0	75.8	75.7	75.5	75.4	75.3	75.1	75.1	75.0	
76						80.2	79.3	78.5	78.1	77.9	77.6	77.4	77.2	77.0	76.8	76.7	76.5	76.5	76.4	76.3	76.2	76.0	
77							80.4	79.5	79.1	78.9	78.6	78.4	78.2	78.0	77.9	77.7	77.5	77.5	77.4	77.3	77.2	77.0	
78								80.6	80.2	79.9	79.6	79.4	79.2	79.0	78.9	78.7	78.5	78.5	78.4	78.3	78.2	78.0	

FIG. 78.

*Figures 77-87 are from Bayley, N., and Pinneau, S. R.: J. Pediat. 40:423 (Tables IIA-E and IIIA-F), 1952.

ACCELERATED BOYS — PERCENTAGES AND ESTIMATED MATURE HEIGHTS FOR BOYS WITH SKELETAL AGES ONE YEAR OR MORE ADVANCED OVER THEIR CHRONOLOGIC AGES

Skeletal Ages 7 through 11 Years

Skeletal Age	7-0	7-3	7-6	7-9	8-0	8-3	8-6	8-9	9-0	9-3	9-6	9-9	10-0	10-3	10-6	10-9	11-0	11-3	11-6	11-9
% of Mature Height	67.0	67.6	68.3	68.9	69.6	70.3	70.9	71.5	72.0	72.8	73.4	74.1	74.7	75.3	75.8	76.3	76.7	77.6	78.6	80.0
Ht. (inches)																				
41	61.2	60.7	60.0																	
42	62.7	62.1	61.5	61.0	60.3															
43	64.2	63.6	63.0	62.4	61.8	61.2	60.6	60.1												
44	65.7	65.1	64.4	63.9	63.2	62.6	62.1	61.5	61.1	60.4										
45	67.2	66.6	65.9	65.3	64.7	64.0	63.5	62.9	62.5	61.8	61.3	60.7	60.2							
46	68.7	68.0	67.3	66.8	66.1	65.4	64.9	64.3	63.9	63.2	62.7	62.1	61.6	61.1	60.7	60.3	60.0			
47	70.1	69.5	68.8	68.2	67.5	66.9	66.3	65.7	65.3	64.6	64.0	63.4	62.9	62.4	62.0	61.6	61.3	60.6		
48	71.6	71.0	70.3	69.7	69.0	68.3	67.7	67.1	66.7	65.9	65.4	64.8	64.3	63.7	63.3	62.9	62.6	61.9	61.1	60.0
49	73.1	72.5	71.7	71.1	70.4	69.7	69.1	68.5	68.1	67.3	66.8	66.1	65.6	65.1	64.6	64.2	63.9	63.1	62.3	61.3
50	74.6	74.0	73.2	72.6	71.8	71.1	70.5	69.9	69.4	68.7	68.1	67.5	66.9	66.4	66.0	65.5	65.2	64.4	63.6	62.5
51	76.2	75.4	74.7	74.0	73.3	72.5	71.9	71.3	70.8	70.1	69.5	68.8	68.3	67.7	67.3	66.8	66.5	65.7	64.9	63.8
52	77.6	76.9	76.1	75.5	74.7	74.0	73.3	72.7	72.2	71.4	70.8	70.2	69.6	69.1	68.6	68.2	67.8	67.0	66.2	65.0
53	79.1	78.4	77.6	76.9	76.2	75.4	74.8	74.1	73.6	72.8	72.2	71.5	71.0	70.4	69.9	69.5	69.1	68.3	67.4	66.3
54	80.6	79.9	79.1	78.4	77.6	76.8	76.2	75.5	75.0	74.2	73.6	72.9	72.3	71.7	71.2	70.8	70.4	69.6	68.7	67.5
55			80.5	79.8	79.0	78.2	77.6	76.9	76.4	75.5	74.9	74.2	73.6	73.0	72.6	72.1	71.7	70.9	70.0	68.8
56					80.5	79.7	79.0	78.3	77.8	76.9	76.3	75.6	75.0	74.4	73.9	73.4	73.0	72.2	71.2	70.0
57							80.4	79.7	79.2	78.3	77.7	76.9	76.3	75.7	75.2	74.7	74.3	73.5	72.5	71.3
58									80.6	79.7	79.0	78.3	77.6	77.0	76.5	76.0	75.6	74.7	73.8	72.5
59											80.4	79.6	79.0	78.4	77.8	77.3	76.9	76.0	75.1	73.8
60													80.3	79.7	79.2	78.6	78.2	77.3	76.3	75.0
61															80.5	79.9	79.5	78.6	77.6	76.3
62																81.3	80.8	79.9	78.9	77.5
63																			80.2	78.8
64																				80.0

FIG. 79.

ACCELERATED BOYS — PERCENTAGES AND ESTIMATED MATURE HEIGHTS FOR BOYS WITH SKELETAL AGES ONE YEAR OR MORE ADVANCED OVER THEIR CHRONOLOGIC AGES

Skeletal Ages 12 through 17 Years

Skeletal Age	12-0	12-3	12-6	12-9	13-0	13-3	13-6	13-9	14-0	14-3	14-6	14-9	15-0	15-3	15-6	15-9	16-0	16-3	16-6	16-9	17-0
% of Mature Height	80.9	81.8	82.8	83.9	85.0	86.3	87.5	89.0	90.5	91.8	93.0	94.3	95.8	96.7	97.1	97.6	98.0	98.3	98.5	98.8	99.0
Ht. (inches)																					
49	60.6																				
50	61.8	61.1	60.4																		
51	63.0	62.3	61.6	60.8	60.0																
52	64.3	63.6	62.8	62.0	61.2	60.3															
53	65.5	64.8	64.0	63.2	62.4	61.4	60.6														
54	66.7	66.0	65.2	64.4	63.5	62.6	61.7	60.7													
55	68.0	67.2	66.4	65.6	64.7	63.7	62.9	61.8	60.8												
56	69.2	68.5	67.6	66.7	65.9	64.9	64.0	62.9	61.9	61.0	60.2										
57	70.5	69.7	68.8	67.9	67.1	66.0	65.1	64.0	63.0	62.1	61.3	60.4									
58	71.7	70.9	70.0	69.1	68.2	67.2	66.3	65.2	64.1	63.2	62.4	61.5	60.5	60.0							
59	72.9	72.1	71.3	70.3	69.4	68.4	67.4	66.3	65.2	64.3	63.4	62.6	61.6	61.0	60.8	60.5	60.2	60.0			
60	74.2	73.4	72.5	71.5	70.6	69.5	68.6	67.4	66.3	65.4	64.5	63.6	62.6	62.0	61.8	61.5	61.2	61.0	60.9	60.7	60.6
61	75.4	74.6	73.7	72.7	71.8	70.7	69.7	68.5	67.4	66.4	65.6	64.7	63.7	63.1	62.8	62.5	62.2	62.1	61.9	61.7	61.6
62	76.6	75.8	74.9	73.9	72.9	71.8	70.9	69.7	68.5	67.5	66.7	65.7	64.7	64.1	63.9	63.5	63.3	63.1	62.9	62.8	62.6
63	77.9	77.0	76.1	75.1	74.1	73.0	72.0	70.8	69.6	68.6	67.7	66.8	65.8	65.1	64.9	64.5	64.3	64.1	64.0	63.8	63.6
64	79.1	78.2	77.3	76.3	75.3	74.2	73.1	71.9	70.7	69.7	68.8	67.9	66.8	66.2	65.9	65.6	65.3	65.1	65.0	64.8	64.6
65	80.3	79.5	78.5	77.5	76.5	75.3	74.3	73.0	71.8	70.8	69.9	68.9	67.8	67.2	66.9	66.6	66.3	66.1	66.0	65.8	65.7
66		80.7	79.7	78.7	77.6	76.5	75.4	74.2	72.9	71.9	71.0	70.0	68.9	68.3	68.0	67.6	67.3	67.1	67.0	66.8	66.7
67			80.9	79.9	78.8	77.6	76.6	75.3	74.0	73.0	72.0	71.1	69.9	69.3	69.0	68.6	68.4	68.2	68.0	67.8	67.7
68					80.0	78.8	77.7	76.4	75.1	74.1	73.1	72.1	71.0	70.3	70.0	69.7	69.4	69.2	69.0	68.8	68.7
69						80.0	78.9	77.5	76.2	75.2	74.2	73.2	72.0	71.4	71.1	70.7	70.4	70.2	70.0	69.8	69.7
70							80.0	78.7	77.3	76.3	75.3	74.2	73.1	72.4	72.1	71.7	71.4	71.2	71.1	70.8	70.7
71								79.8	78.5	77.3	76.3	75.3	74.1	73.4	73.1	72.7	72.4	72.2	72.1	71.9	71.7
72								80.9	79.6	78.4	77.4	76.4	75.2	74.5	74.2	73.8	73.5	73.2	73.1	72.9	72.7
73									80.7	79.5	78.5	77.4	76.2	75.5	75.2	74.8	74.5	74.3	74.1	73.9	73.7
74										80.6	79.6	78.5	77.2	76.5	76.2	75.8	75.5	75.3	75.1	74.9	74.7
75											80.6	79.5	78.3	77.6	77.2	76.8	76.5	76.3	76.1	75.9	75.8
76												80.4	79.3	78.6	78.3	77.9	77.6	77.3	77.2	76.9	76.8
77													80.4	79.6	79.3	78.9	78.6	78.3	78.2	77.9	77.8
78														80.7	80.3	79.9	79.6	79.3	79.2	78.9	78.8

FIG. 80.

RETARDED BOYS — PERCENTAGES AND ESTIMATED MATURE HEIGHTS FOR BOYS WITH SKELETAL AGES ONE YEAR OR MORE RETARDED FOR THEIR CHRONOLOGIC AGES

Skeletal Ages 6 through 13 Years

Skeletal Age / Ht. (inches)	6-0	6-3	6-6	6-9	7-0	7-3	7-6	7-9	8-0	8-3	8-6	8-9	9-0	9-3	9-6	9-9	10-0	10-3	10-6	10-9	11-0	11-3	11-6	11-9	12-0	12-3	12-6	12-9	13-0
% of Mature Height	68.0	69.0	70.0	70.9	71.8	72.8	73.8	74.7	75.6	76.5	77.3	77.9	78.6	79.4	80.0	80.7	81.2	81.6	81.9	82.1	82.3	82.7	83.2	83.9	84.5	85.2	86.0	86.9	88.0
41	60.3																												
42	61.8	60.9	60.0																										
43	63.2	62.3	61.4	60.6																									
44	64.7	63.8	62.9	62.1	61.3	60.4																							
45	66.2	65.2	64.3	63.5	62.7	61.8	61.0	60.2																					
46	67.6	66.7	65.7	64.9	64.1	63.2	62.3	61.6	60.8	60.1																			
47	69.1	68.1	67.1	66.3	65.5	64.6	63.7	62.9	62.2	61.4	60.8	60.1																	
48	70.6	69.6	68.6	67.7	66.9	65.9	65.0	64.3	63.5	62.7	62.1	61.6	61.1	60.5	60.0														
49	72.1	71.0	70.0	69.1	68.3	67.3	66.4	65.6	64.8	64.1	63.4	62.9	62.3	61.7	61.3	60.7	60.3	60.0											
50	73.5	72.5	71.4	70.5	69.6	68.7	67.8	66.9	66.1	65.4	64.7	64.2	63.6	63.0	62.5	62.0	61.6	61.3	61.1	60.9	60.8	60.5	60.1						
51	75.0	73.9	72.9	71.9	71.0	70.1	69.1	68.3	67.5	66.7	66.0	65.5	64.9	64.2	63.8	63.2	62.8	62.5	62.3	62.1	62.0	61.7	61.3	60.8	60.4				
52	76.5	75.4	74.3	73.3	72.4	71.4	70.5	69.6	68.8	68.0	67.3	66.8	66.2	65.5	65.0	64.4	64.0	63.7	63.5	63.3	63.2	62.9	62.5	62.0	61.5	61.0	60.5		
53	77.9	76.8	75.7	74.8	73.8	72.8	71.8	71.0	70.1	69.3	68.6	68.0	67.4	66.8	66.3	65.7	65.3	65.0	64.7	64.6	64.4	64.1	63.7	63.2	62.7	62.2	61.6	61.0	60.2
54	79.4	78.3	77.1	76.2	75.2	74.2	73.2	72.3	71.4	70.6	69.9	69.3	68.7	68.0	67.5	66.9	66.5	66.2	65.9	65.8	65.6	65.3	64.9	64.4	63.9	63.4	62.8	62.1	61.4
55	80.9	79.7	78.6	77.6	76.6	75.5	74.5	73.6	72.8	71.9	71.2	70.6	70.0	69.3	68.8	68.2	67.7	67.4	67.2	67.0	66.8	66.5	66.1	65.6	65.1	64.6	64.0	63.3	62.5
56		80.0	79.0	78.0	76.9	75.9	75.0	74.1	73.2	72.4	71.9	71.2	70.5	70.0	69.4	69.0	68.6	68.4	68.2	68.0	67.7	67.3	66.7	66.3	65.7	65.1	64.4	63.6	
57				80.4	79.4	78.3	77.2	76.3	75.4	74.5	73.7	73.2	72.5	71.8	71.3	70.6	70.2	69.9	69.6	69.4	69.3	68.9	68.5	67.9	67.5	66.9	66.3	65.6	64.8
58					80.8	79.7	78.6	77.6	76.7	75.8	75.0	74.5	73.8	73.0	72.5	71.9	71.4	71.1	70.8	70.6	70.5	70.1	69.7	69.1	68.6	68.1	67.4	66.7	65.9
59							79.9	79.0	78.0	77.1	76.3	75.7	75.1	74.3	73.8	73.1	72.7	72.3	72.0	71.9	71.7	71.3	70.9	70.3	69.8	69.2	68.6	67.9	67.0
60								80.3	79.4	78.4	77.6	77.0	76.3	75.6	75.0	74.4	73.9	73.5	73.3	73.1	72.9	72.6	72.1	71.5	71.0	70.4	69.8	69.0	68.2
61									80.7	79.7	78.9	78.3	77.6	76.8	76.3	75.6	75.1	74.8	74.5	74.3	74.1	73.8	73.3	72.7	72.2	71.6	70.9	70.2	69.3
62											80.2	79.6	78.9	78.1	77.5	76.8	76.4	76.0	75.7	75.5	75.3	75.0	74.5	73.9	73.4	72.8	72.1	71.3	70.5
63												80.9	80.2	79.3	78.8	78.1	77.6	77.2	76.9	76.7	76.5	76.2	75.7	75.1	74.6	73.9	73.3	72.5	71.6
64														80.6	80.0	79.3	78.8	78.4	78.1	78.0	77.8	77.4	76.9	76.3	75.7	75.1	74.4	73.6	72.7
65																80.5	80.0	79.7	79.4	79.2	79.0	78.6	78.1	77.5	76.9	76.3	75.6	74.8	73.9
66																		80.9	80.6	80.4	80.2	79.8	79.3	78.7	78.1	77.5	76.7	75.9	75.0
67																							80.5	79.9	79.3	78.6	77.9	77.1	76.1

FIG. 81.

AVERAGE GIRLS — PERCENTAGES AND ESTIMATED MATURE HEIGHTS FOR GIRLS WITH SKELETAL AGES WITHIN ONE YEAR OF THEIR CHRONOLOGIC AGES

Skeletal Ages 6 through 11 Years

Skeletal Age / Ht. (inches)	6-0	6-3	6-6	6-10	7-0	7-3	7-6	7-10	8-0	8-3	8-6	8-10	9-0	9-3	9-6	9-9	10-0	10-3	10-6	10-9	11-0	11-3	11-6	11-9
% of Mature Height	72.0	72.9	73.8	75.1	75.7	76.5	77.2	78.2	79.0	80.1	81.0	82.1	82.7	83.6	84.4	85.3	86.2	87.4	88.4	89.6	90.6	91.0	91.4	91.8
37	51.4																							
38	52.8	52.1	51.5																					
39	54.2	53.5	52.8	52.0	51.5	51.0																		
40	55.6	54.9	54.2	53.3	52.8	52.3	51.8	51.2																
41	56.9	56.2	55.6	54.6	54.2	53.6	53.1	52.4	51.9	51.2														
42	58.3	57.6	56.9	55.9	55.5	54.9	54.4	53.7	53.2	52.4	51.9	51.2												
43	59.7	59.0	58.3	57.3	56.8	56.2	55.7	55.0	54.4	53.7	53.1	52.4	52.0	51.4										
44	61.1	60.4	59.6	58.6	58.1	57.5	57.0	56.3	55.7	54.9	54.3	53.6	53.2	52.6	52.1	51.6	51.0							
45	62.5	61.7	61.0	59.9	59.4	58.8	58.3	57.5	57.0	56.2	55.6	54.8	54.4	53.8	53.3	52.8	52.2	51.5						
46	63.9	63.1	62.3	61.3	60.8	60.1	59.6	58.8	58.2	57.4	56.8	56.0	55.5	55.0	54.5	53.9	53.4	52.6	52.0	51.3				
47	65.3	64.5	63.7	62.6	62.1	61.4	60.9	60.1	59.5	58.7	58.0	57.2	56.8	56.2	55.7	55.1	54.5	53.8	53.2	52.5	51.9	51.6	51.4	51.2
48	66.7	65.8	65.0	63.9	63.4	62.7	62.2	61.4	60.8	59.9	59.3	58.5	58.0	57.4	56.9	56.3	55.7	54.9	54.3	53.6	53.0	52.7	52.5	52.3
49	68.1	67.2	66.4	65.2	64.7	64.1	63.5	62.7	62.0	61.2	60.5	59.7	59.3	58.6	58.1	57.4	56.8	56.1	55.4	54.7	54.1	53.8	53.6	53.4
50	69.4	68.6	67.8	66.6	66.1	65.4	64.8	63.9	63.3	62.4	61.7	60.9	60.5	59.8	59.2	58.6	58.0	57.2	56.6	55.8	55.2	54.9	54.7	54.5
51	70.8	70.0	69.1	67.9	67.4	66.7	66.1	65.2	64.6	63.7	63.0	62.1	61.7	61.0	60.4	59.8	59.2	58.4	57.7	56.9	56.3	56.0	55.8	55.6
52	72.2	71.3	70.5	69.2	68.7	68.0	67.4	66.5	65.8	64.9	64.2	63.3	62.9	62.2	61.6	61.0	60.3	59.5	58.8	58.0	57.4	57.1	56.9	56.6
53	73.6	72.7	71.8	70.6	70.0	69.3	68.7	67.8	67.1	66.2	65.4	64.6	64.1	63.4	62.8	62.1	61.5	60.6	60.0	59.2	58.5	58.2	58.0	57.7
54		74.1	73.2	71.9	71.3	70.6	70.0	69.1	68.4	67.4	66.7	65.8	65.3	64.6	64.0	63.3	62.6	61.8	61.1	60.3	59.6	59.3	59.1	58.8
55			74.5	73.2	72.7	71.9	71.2	70.3	69.6	68.7	67.9	67.0	66.5	65.8	65.2	64.5	63.8	62.9	62.2	61.4	60.7	60.4	60.2	59.9
56				74.6	74.0	73.2	72.5	71.6	70.9	69.9	69.1	68.2	67.7	67.0	66.4	65.7	65.0	64.1	63.3	62.5	61.8	61.5	61.3	61.0
57						74.5	73.8	72.9	72.2	71.2	70.4	69.4	68.9	68.2	67.5	66.8	66.1	65.2	64.5	63.6	62.9	62.6	62.4	62.1
58								74.2	73.4	72.4	71.6	70.6	70.1	69.4	68.7	68.0	67.3	66.4	65.6	64.7	64.0	63.7	63.5	63.2
59									74.7	73.7	72.8	71.9	71.3	70.6	69.9	69.2	68.4	67.5	66.7	65.8	65.1	64.8	64.6	64.3
60										74.9	74.1	73.1	72.6	71.8	71.1	70.3	69.6	68.7	67.9	67.0	66.2	65.9	65.6	65.4
61												74.3	73.8	73.0	72.3	71.5	70.8	69.8	69.0	68.1	67.3	67.0	66.7	66.4
62														74.2	73.5	72.7	71.9	70.9	70.1	69.2	68.4	68.1	67.8	67.5
63															74.6	73.9	73.1	72.1	71.3	70.3	69.5	69.2	68.9	68.6
64																	74.2	73.2	72.4	71.4	70.6	70.3	70.0	69.7
65																		74.4	73.5	72.5	71.7	71.4	71.1	70.8
66																			74.7	73.7	72.9	72.5	72.2	71.9
67																				74.8	74.0	73.6	73.3	73.0
68																						74.7	74.4	74.1

FIG. 82.

PREDICTION OF ADULT HEIGHT FROM SKELETAL AGE

AVERAGE GIRLS — PERCENTAGES AND ESTIMATED MATURE HEIGHTS FOR GIRLS WITH SKELETAL AGES WITHIN ONE YEAR OF THEIR CHRONOLOGIC AGES

Skeletal Ages 12 through 18 Years

Skeletal Age	12-0	12-3	12-6	12-9	13-0	13-3	13-6	13-9	14-0	14-3	14-6	14-9	15-0	15-3	15-6	15-9	16-0	16-3	16-6	16-9	17-0	17-6	18-0
% of Mature Height / Ht. (inches)	92.2	93.2	94.1	95.0	95.8	96.7	97.4	97.8	98.0	98.3	98.6	98.8	99.0	99.1	99.3	99.4	99.6	99.6	99.7	99.8	99.9	99.95	100.0
47	51.0																						
48	52.1	51.5	51.0																				
49	53.1	52.6	52.1	51.6	51.1																		
50	54.2	53.6	53.1	52.6	52.2	51.7	51.3	51.1	51.0														
51	55.3	54.7	54.2	53.7	53.2	52.7	52.4	52.1	52.0	51.9	51.7	51.6	51.5	51.5	51.4	51.3	51.2	51.2	51.2	51.1	51.1	51.0	51.0
52	56.4	55.8	55.3	54.7	54.3	53.8	53.4	53.2	53.1	52.9	52.7	52.6	52.5	52.5	52.4	52.3	52.2	52.2	52.2	52.1	52.1	52.0	52.0
53	57.5	56.9	56.3	55.8	55.3	54.8	54.4	54.2	54.1	53.9	53.8	53.6	53.5	53.5	53.4	53.3	53.2	53.2	53.2	53.1	53.1	53.0	53.0
54	58.6	57.9	57.4	56.8	56.4	55.8	55.4	55.2	55.1	54.9	54.8	54.7	54.5	54.5	54.4	54.3	54.2	54.2	54.2	54.1	54.1	54.0	54.0
55	59.7	59.0	58.4	57.9	57.4	56.9	56.5	56.2	56.1	56.0	55.8	55.7	55.6	55.5	55.4	55.3	55.2	55.2	55.2	55.1	55.1	55.0	55.0
56	60.7	60.1	59.5	58.9	58.5	57.9	57.5	57.3	57.1	57.0	56.8	56.7	56.6	56.5	56.4	56.3	56.2	56.2	56.2	56.1	56.1	56.0	56.0
57	61.8	61.2	60.6	60.0	59.5	58.9	58.5	58.3	58.2	58.0	57.8	57.7	57.6	57.5	57.4	57.3	57.2	57.2	57.2	57.1	57.1	57.0	57.0
58	62.9	62.2	61.6	61.1	60.5	60.0	59.5	59.3	59.2	59.0	58.8	58.7	58.6	58.5	58.4	58.3	58.2	58.2	58.2	58.1	58.1	58.0	58.0
59	64.0	63.3	62.7	62.1	61.6	61.0	60.6	60.3	60.2	60.0	59.8	59.7	59.6	59.5	59.4	59.4	59.2	59.2	59.2	59.1	59.1	59.0	59.0
60	65.1	64.4	63.8	63.2	62.6	62.0	61.6	61.3	61.2	61.0	60.9	60.7	60.6	60.5	60.4	60.4	60.2	60.2	60.2	60.1	60.1	60.0	60.0
61	66.2	65.5	64.8	64.2	63.7	63.1	62.6	62.4	62.2	62.1	61.9	61.7	61.6	61.6	61.4	61.4	61.2	61.2	61.2	61.1	61.1	61.0	61.0
62	67.2	66.5	65.9	65.3	64.7	64.1	63.7	63.4	63.3	63.1	62.9	62.8	62.6	62.6	62.4	62.4	62.2	62.2	62.2	62.1	62.1	62.0	62.0
63	68.3	67.6	67.0	66.3	65.8	65.1	64.7	64.4	64.3	64.1	63.9	63.8	63.6	63.6	63.4	63.4	63.3	63.3	63.2	63.1	63.1	63.0	63.0
64	69.4	68.7	68.0	67.4	66.8	66.2	65.7	65.4	65.3	65.1	64.9	64.8	64.6	64.6	64.4	64.4	64.3	64.3	64.2	64.1	64.1	64.0	64.0
65	70.5	69.7	69.1	68.4	67.8	67.2	66.7	66.5	66.3	66.1	65.9	65.8	65.7	65.6	65.5	65.4	65.3	65.3	65.2	65.1	65.1	65.0	65.0
66	71.6	70.8	70.1	69.5	68.9	68.3	67.8	67.5	67.3	67.1	66.9	66.8	66.7	66.6	66.5	66.4	66.3	66.3	66.2	66.1	66.1	66.0	66.0
67	72.7	71.9	71.2	70.5	69.9	69.3	68.8	68.5	68.4	68.2	68.0	67.8	67.7	67.6	67.5	67.4	67.3	67.3	67.2	67.1	67.1	67.0	67.0
68	73.8	73.0	72.3	71.6	71.0	70.3	69.8	69.5	69.4	69.2	69.0	68.8	68.7	68.6	68.5	68.4	68.3	68.3	68.2	68.1	68.1	68.0	68.0
69	74.8	74.0	73.3	72.6	72.0	71.4	70.8	70.6	70.4	70.2	70.0	69.8	69.7	69.6	69.5	69.4	69.3	69.3	69.2	69.1	69.1	69.0	69.0
70			74.4	73.7	73.1	72.4	71.9	71.6	71.4	71.2	71.0	70.8	70.7	70.6	70.5	70.4	70.3	70.3	70.2	70.1	70.1	70.0	70.0
71				74.7	74.1	73.4	72.9	72.6	72.4	72.2	72.0	71.9	71.7	71.6	71.5	71.4	71.3	71.3	71.2	71.1	71.1	71.0	71.0
72						74.5	73.9	73.6	73.5	73.2	73.0	72.9	72.7	72.7	72.5	72.4	72.3	72.3	72.2	72.1	72.1	72.0	72.0
73							74.9	74.6	74.5	74.3	74.0	73.9	73.7	73.7	73.5	73.4	73.3	73.3	73.2	73.1	73.1	73.0	73.0
74												74.9	74.7	74.7	74.5	74.4	74.3	74.3	74.2	74.1	74.1	74.0	74.0

FIG. 83.

ACCELERATED GIRLS — PERCENTAGES AND ESTIMATED MATURE HEIGHTS FOR GIRLS WITH SKELETAL AGES ONE YEAR OR MORE ADVANCED OVER THEIR CHRONOLOGIC AGES

Skeletal Ages 7 through 11 Years

Skeletal Age	7-0	7-3	7-6	7-10	8-0	8-3	8-6	8-10	9-0	9-3	9-6	9-9	10-0	10-3	10-6	10-9	11-0	11-3	11-6	11-9
% of Mature Height / Ht. (inches)	71.2	72.2	73.2	74.2	75.0	76.0	77.1	78.4	79.0	80.0	80.9	81.9	82.8	84.1	85.6	87.0	88.3	88.7	89.1	89.7
37	52.0	51.2																		
38	53.4	52.6	51.9	51.2																
39	54.8	54.0	53.3	52.6	52.0	51.3														
40	56.2	55.4	54.6	53.9	53.3	52.6	51.9	51.0												
41	57.6	56.8	56.0	55.3	54.7	53.9	53.2	52.3	51.9	51.3										
42	59.0	58.2	57.4	56.6	56.0	55.3	54.5	53.6	53.2	52.5	51.9	51.3								
43	60.4	59.6	58.7	58.0	57.3	56.6	55.8	54.8	54.4	53.8	53.2	52.5	51.9	51.1						
44	61.8	60.9	60.1	59.3	58.7	57.9	57.1	56.1	55.7	55.0	54.4	53.7	53.1	52.3	51.4					
45	63.2	62.3	61.5	60.6	60.0	59.2	58.4	57.4	57.0	56.3	55.6	54.9	54.3	53.5	52.6	51.7	51.0			
46	64.6	63.7	62.8	62.0	61.3	60.5	59.7	58.7	58.2	57.5	56.9	56.2	55.6	54.7	53.7	52.9	52.1	51.9	51.6	51.3
47	66.0	65.1	64.2	63.3	62.7	61.8	61.0	59.9	59.5	58.8	58.1	57.4	56.8	55.9	54.9	54.0	53.2	53.0	52.7	52.4
48	67.4	66.5	65.6	64.7	64.0	63.2	62.3	61.2	60.8	60.0	59.3	58.6	58.0	57.1	56.1	55.2	54.4	54.1	53.9	53.5
49	68.8	67.9	66.9	66.0	65.3	64.5	63.6	62.5	62.0	61.3	60.6	59.8	59.2	58.3	57.2	56.3	55.5	55.2	55.0	54.6
50	70.2	69.3	68.3	67.4	66.7	65.8	64.9	63.8	63.3	62.5	61.8	61.1	60.4	59.5	58.4	57.5	56.6	56.4	56.1	55.7
51	71.6	70.6	69.7	68.7	68.0	67.1	66.1	65.1	64.6	63.8	63.0	62.3	61.6	60.6	59.6	58.6	57.8	57.5	57.2	56.9
52	73.0	72.0	71.0	70.1	69.3	68.4	67.4	66.3	65.8	65.0	64.3	63.5	62.8	61.8	60.7	59.8	58.9	58.6	58.4	58.0
53	74.4	73.4	72.4	71.4	70.7	69.7	68.7	67.6	67.1	66.3	65.5	64.7	64.0	63.0	61.9	60.9	60.0	59.8	59.5	59.1
54		74.8	73.8	72.8	72.0	71.1	70.0	68.9	68.4	67.5	66.7	65.9	65.2	64.2	63.1	62.1	61.2	60.9	60.6	60.2
55				74.1	73.3	72.4	71.3	70.2	69.6	68.8	68.0	67.2	66.4	65.4	64.3	63.2	62.3	62.0	61.7	61.3
56					74.7	73.7	72.6	71.4	70.9	70.0	69.2	68.4	67.6	66.6	65.4	64.4	63.4	63.1	62.8	62.4
57							73.9	72.7	72.2	71.3	70.5	69.6	68.8	67.8	66.6	65.5	64.6	64.3	64.0	63.5
58								74.0	73.4	72.5	71.7	70.8	70.0	69.0	67.8	66.7	65.7	65.4	65.1	64.7
59									74.7	73.8	72.9	72.0	71.3	70.2	68.9	67.8	66.8	66.5	66.2	65.8
60											74.2	73.3	72.5	71.3	70.1	69.0	68.0	67.6	67.3	66.9
61												74.5	73.7	72.5	71.3	70.1	69.1	68.8	68.5	68.0
62													74.9	73.7	72.4	71.3	70.2	69.9	69.6	69.1
63														74.9	73.6	72.4	71.3	71.0	70.7	70.2
64															74.8	73.6	72.5	72.2	71.8	71.3
65																74.7	73.6	73.3	72.9	72.5
66																	74.7	74.4	74.1	73.6
67																				74.7

FIG. 84.

ACCELERATED GIRLS — PERCENTAGES AND ESTIMATED MATURE HEIGHTS FOR GIRLS WITH SKELETAL AGES ONE YEAR OR MORE ADVANCED OVER THEIR CHRONOLOGIC AGES

Skeletal Ages 12 through 17 Years

Skeletal Age	12-0	12-3	12-6	12-9	13-0	13-3	13-6	13-9	14-0	14-3	14-6	14-9	15-0	15-3	15-6	15-9	16-0	16-3	16-6	16-9	17-0	17-6
% of Mature Height	90.1	91.3	92.4	93.5	94.5	95.5	96.3	96.8	97.2	97.7	98.0	98.3	98.6	98.8	99.0	99.2	99.3	99.4	99.5	99.7	99.8	99.95
Ht. (inches)																						
46	51.1																					
47	52.2	51.5																				
48	53.3	52.6	51.9	51.3																		
49	54.4	53.7	53.0	52.4	51.9	51.3	50.9															
50	55.5	54.8	54.1	53.5	52.9	52.4	51.9	51.7	51.4	51.2	51.0											
51	56.6	55.9	55.2	54.5	54.0	53.4	53.0	52.7	52.5	52.2	52.0	51.9	51.7	51.6	51.5	51.4	51.4	51.3	51.3	51.2	51.1	51.0
52	57.7	57.0	56.3	55.6	55.0	54.5	54.0	53.7	53.5	53.2	53.1	52.9	52.7	52.6	52.5	52.4	52.4	52.3	52.3	52.2	52.1	52.0
53	58.8	58.1	57.4	56.7	56.1	55.5	55.0	54.8	54.5	54.2	54.1	53.9	53.8	53.6	53.5	53.4	53.4	53.3	53.3	53.2	53.1	53.0
54	59.9	59.1	58.4	57.8	57.1	56.5	56.1	55.8	55.6	55.3	55.1	54.9	54.8	54.7	54.5	54.4	54.4	54.3	54.3	54.2	54.1	54.0
55	61.0	60.2	59.5	58.8	58.2	57.6	57.1	56.8	56.6	56.3	56.1	56.0	55.8	55.7	55.5	55.4	55.4	55.3	55.3	55.2	55.1	55.0
56	62.2	61.3	60.6	59.9	59.3	58.6	58.2	57.9	57.6	57.3	57.1	57.0	56.8	56.7	56.5	56.5	56.4	56.3	56.2	56.1	56.0	
57	63.3	62.4	61.7	61.0	60.3	59.7	59.2	58.9	58.6	58.3	58.2	58.0	57.8	57.7	57.6	57.5	57.4	57.3	57.3	57.2	57.1	57.0
58	64.4	63.5	62.8	62.0	61.4	60.7	60.2	59.9	59.7	59.4	59.2	59.0	58.8	58.7	58.6	58.5	58.4	58.3	58.3	58.2	58.1	58.0
59	6.55	64.6	63.9	63.1	62.4	61.8	61.3	61.0	60.7	60.4	60.2	60.0	59.8	59.7	59.6	59.5	59.4	59.4	59.3	59.2	59.1	59.0
60	66.6	65.7	64.9	64.2	63.5	62.8	62.3	62.0	61.7	61.4	61.2	61.0	60.9	60.7	60.6	60.5	60.4	60.4	60.3	60.2	60.1	60.0
61	67.7	66.8	66.0	65.2	64.6	63.9	63.3	63.0	62.8	62.4	62.2	62.1	61.9	61.7	61.6	61.5	61.4	61.4	61.3	61.2	61.1	61.0
62	68.8	67.9	67.1	66.3	65.6	64.9	64.4	64.0	63.8	63.5	63.3	63.1	62.9	62.8	62.6	62.5	62.4	62.4	62.3	62.2	62.1	62.0
63	69.9	69.0	68.2	67.4	66.7	66.0	65.4	65.1	64.8	64.5	64.3	64.1	63.9	63.8	63.6	63.5	63.4	63.4	63.3	63.2	63.1	63.0
64	71.0	70.1	69.3	68.4	67.7	67.0	66.5	66.1	65.8	65.5	65.3	65.1	64.9	64.8	64.6	64.5	64.4	64.4	64.3	64.2	64.1	64.0
65	72.1	71.2	70.3	69.5	68.8	68.1	67.5	67.1	66.9	66.5	66.3	66.1	65.9	65.8	65.7	65.5	65.5	65.4	65.3	65.2	65.1	65.0
66	73.3	72.3	71.4	70.6	69.8	69.1	68.5	68.2	67.9	67.6	67.3	67.1	66.9	66.8	66.7	66.5	66.5	66.4	66.3	66.2	66.1	66.0
67	74.4	73.4	72.5	71.7	70.9	70.2	69.6	69.2	68.9	68.6	68.4	68.2	68.0	67.8	67.7	67.5	67.5	67.4	67.3	67.2	67.1	67.0
68		74.5	73.6	72.7	72.0	71.2	70.6	70.2	70.0	69.6	69.4	69.2	69.0	68.8	68.7	68.6	68.5	68.4	68.3	68.2	68.1	68.0
69			74.7	73.8	73.0	72.3	71.7	71.3	71.0	70.6	70.4	70.2	70.0	69.8	69.7	69.6	69.5	69.4	69.3	69.2	69.1	69.0
70				74.9	74.1	73.3	72.7	72.3	72.0	71.6	71.4	71.2	71.0	70.8	70.7	70.6	70.5	70.4	70.3	70.2	70.1	70.0
71						74.3	73.7	73.3	73.0	72.7	72.4	72.2	72.0	71.9	71.7	71.6	71.5	71.4	71.4	71.2	71.1	71.0
72							74.8	74.4	74.1	73.7	73.5	73.2	73.0	72.9	72.7	72.6	72.5	72.4	72.4	72.2	72.1	72.0
73										74.7	74.5	74.3	74.0	73.9	73.7	73.6	73.5	734.	73.4	73.2	73.1	73.0
74														74.9	74.4	74.6	74.5	74.4	74.4	74.2	74.1	74.0

FIG. 85.

RETARDED GIRLS — PERCENTAGES AND ESTIMATED MATURE HEIGHTS FOR GIRLS WITH SKELETAL AGES ONE YEAR OR MORE RETARDED FOR THEIR CHRONOLOGIC AGES

Skeletal Ages 6 through 11 Years

Skeletal Age	6-0	6-3	6-6	6-10	7-0	7-3	7-6	7-10	8-0	8-3	8-6	8-10	9-0	9-3	9-6	9-9	10-0	10-3	10-6	10-9	11-0	11-3	11-6	11-9
% of Mature Height	73.3	74.2	75.1	76.3	77.0	77.9	78.8	79.7	80.4	81.3	82.3	83.6	84.1	85.1	85.8	86.6	87.4	88.4	89.6	90.7	91.8	92.2	92.6	92.9
Ht. (inches)																								
38	51.8	51.2																						
39	53.2	52.6	51.9	51.1																				
40	54.6	53.9	53.3	52.4	51.9	51.3																		
41	55.9	55.3	54.6	53.7	53.2	52.6	52.0	51.4																
42	57.3	56.6	55.9	55.0	54.5	53.9	53.3	52.7	52.2	51.7	51.0													
43	58.7	58.0	57.3	56.4	55.8	55.2	54.6	54.0	53.5	52.9	52.2	51.4	51.1											
44	60.0	59.3	58.6	57.7	57.1	56.5	55.8	55.2	54.7	54.1	53.5	52.6	52.3	51.7	51.3									
45	61.4	60.6	59.9	59.0	58.4	57.8	57.1	56.5	56.0	55.4	54.7	53.8	53.5	52.9	52.4	52.0	51.5							
46	62.8	62.0	61.3	60.3	59.7	59.1	58.4	57.7	57.2	56.6	55.9	55.0	54.7	54.1	53.6	53.1	52.6	52.0	51.3					
47	64.1	63.3	62.6	61.6	61.0	60.3	59.6	59.0	58.5	57.8	57.1	56.2	55.9	55.2	54.8	54.3	53.8	53.2	52.5	51.8	51.2	51.0		
48	65.5	64.7	63.9	62.9	62.3	61.6	60.9	60.2	59.7	59.0	58.3	57.4	57.1	56.4	55.9	55.4	54.9	54.3	53.6	52.9	52.3	52.1	51.8	51.7
49	66.9	66.0	65.2	64.2	63.6	62.9	62.2	61.5	60.9	60.3	59.5	58.6	58.3	57.6	57.1	56.6	56.1	55.4	54.7	54.0	53.4	53.1	52.9	52.7
50	68.2	67.4	66.6	65.5	64.9	64.2	63.5	62.7	62.2	61.5	60.8	59.8	59.5	58.8	58.3	57.7	57.2	56.6	55.8	55.1	54.5	54.2	54.0	53.8
51	69.6	68.7	67.9	66.8	66.2	65.5	64.7	64.0	63.4	62.7	62.0	61.0	60.6	59.9	59.4	58.9	58.4	57.7	56.9	56.2	55.6	55.3	55.1	54.9
52	70.9	70.1	69.2	68.2	67.5	66.8	66.0	65.2	64.7	64.0	63.2	62.2	61.8	61.1	60.6	60.0	59.5	58.8	58.0	57.3	56.6	56.4	56.2	56.0
53	72.3	71.4	70.6	69.5	68.8	68.0	67.3	66.5	65.9	65.2	64.4	63.4	63.0	62.3	61.8	61.2	60.6	60.0	59.2	58.4	57.7	57.5	57.2	57.1
54	73.7	72.8	71.9	70.8	70.1	69.3	68.5	67.8	67.2	66.4	65.6	64.6	64.2	63.5	62.9	62.4	61.8	61.1	60.3	59.5	58.8	58.6	58.3	58.1
55		74.1	73.2	72.1	71.4	70.6	69.8	69.0	68.4	67.7	66.8	65.8	65.4	64.6	64.1	63.5	62.9	62.2	61.4	60.6	59.9	59.7	59.4	59.2
56			74.6	73.4	72.7	71.9	71.1	70.3	69.7	68.9	68.0	67.0	66.6	65.8	65.3	64.7	64.1	63.3	62.5	61.7	61.0	60.7	60.5	60.3
57				74.7	74.0	73.2	72.3	71.5	70.9	70.1	69.3	68.2	67.8	67.0	66.4	65.8	65.2	64.5	63.6	62.8	62.1	61.8	61.6	61.4
58						74.5	73.6	72.8	72.1	71.3	70.5	69.4	69.0	68.2	67.6	67.0	66.4	65.6	64.7	63.9	63.2	62.9	62.6	62.4
59							74.9	74.0	73.4	72.6	71.7	70.6	70.2	69.3	68.8	68.1	67.5	66.7	65.8	65.0	64.3	64.0	63.7	63.5
60									74.6	73.8	72.9	71.8	71.3	70.5	69.9	69.3	68.7	67.9	67.0	66.2	65.4	65.1	64.8	64.6
61											74.1	73.0	72.5	71.7	71.1	70.4	69.8	69.0	68.1	67.3	66.4	66.2	65.9	65.7
62												74.2	73.7	72.9	72.3	71.6	70.9	70.1	69.2	68.4	67.5	67.2	67.0	66.7
63													74.7	74.0	73.4	72.7	72.1	71.3	70.3	69.5	68.6	68.3	68.0	67.8
64															74.6	73.9	73.2	72.4	71.4	70.6	69.7	69.4	69.1	68.9
65																	74.4	73.5	72.5	71.7	70.8	70.5	70.2	70.0
66																		74.7	73.7	72.8	71.9	71.6	71.3	71.0
67																			74.8	73.9	73.0	72.7	72.4	72.1
68																					74.1	73.8	73.4	73.2
69																						74.8	74.5	74.3

FIG. 86.

PREDICTION OF ADULT HEIGHT FROM SKELETAL AGE

RETARDED GIRLS — PERCENTAGES AND ESTIMATED MATURE HEIGHTS FOR GIRLS WITH SKELETAL AGES ONE YEAR OR MORE RETARDED FOR THEIR CHRONOLOGIC AGES

Skeletal Ages 12 through 17 Years

Skeletal Age	12-0	12-3	12-6	12-9	13-0	13-3	13-6	13-9	14-0	14-3	14-6	14-9	15-0	15-3	15-6	15-9	16-0	16-3	16-6	16-9	17-0
% of Mature Height — Ht. (inches)	93.2	94.2	94.9	95.7	96.4	97.1	97.7	98.1	98.3	98.6	98.9	99.2	99.4	99.5	99.6	99.7	99.8	99.9	99.9	99.95	100.0
48	51.5	51.0																			
49	52.6	52.0	51.6	51.2																	
50	53.6	53.1	52.7	52.2	51.9	51.5	51.2	51.0													
51	54.7	54.1	53.7	53.3	52.9	52.5	52.2	52.0	51.9	51.7	51.6	51.4	51.3	51.3	51.2	51.2	51.1	51.1	51.1	51.0	51.0
52	55.8	55.2	54.8	54.3	53.9	53.6	53.2	53.0	52.9	52.7	52.6	52.4	52.3	52.3	52.2	52.2	52.1	52.1	52.1	52.0	52.0
53	56.9	56.3	55.8	55.4	55.0	54.6	54.2	54.0	53.9	53.8	53.6	53.4	53.3	53.3	53.2	53.2	53.1	53.1	53.1	53.0	53.0
54	57.9	57.3	56.9	56.4	56.0	55.6	55.3	55.0	54.9	54.8	54.6	54.4	54.3	54.3	54.2	54.2	54.1	54.1	54.1	54.0	54.0
55	59.0	58.4	58.0	57.5	57.1	56.6	56.3	56.1	56.0	55.8	55.6	55.4	55.3	55.3	55.2	55.2	55.1	55.1	55.1	55.0	55.0
56	60.1	59.4	59.0	58.5	58.1	57.7	57.3	57.1	57.0	56.8	56.6	56.5	56.3	56.3	56.2	56.2	56.1	56.1	56.1	56.0	56.0
57	61.2	60.5	60.1	59.6	59.1	58.7	58.3	58.1	58.0	57.8	57.6	57.5	57.3	57.3	57.2	57.2	57.1	57.1	57.1	57.0	57.0
58	62.2	61.6	61.1	60.6	60.2	59.7	59.4	59.1	59.0	58.8	58.6	58.5	58.3	58.3	58.2	58.2	58.1	58.1	58.1	58.0	58.0
59	63.3	62.6	62.2	61.7	61.2	60.8	60.4	60.1	60.0	59.8	59.7	59.5	59.4	59.3	59.2	59.2	59.1	59.1	59.1	59.0	59.0
60	64.4	63.7	63.2	62.7	62.2	61.8	61.4	61.2	61.0	60.9	60.7	60.5	60.4	60.3	60.2	60.2	60.1	60.1	60.1	60.0	60.0
61	65.5	64.8	64.3	63.7	63.3	62.8	62.4	62.2	62.1	61.9	61.7	61.5	61.4	61.3	61.2	61.2	61.1	61.1	61.1	61.0	61.0
62	66.5	65.8	65.3	64.8	64.3	63.9	63.5	63.2	63.1	62.9	62.7	62.5	62.4	62.3	62.2	62.2	62.1	62.1	62.1	62.0	62.0
63	67.6	66.9	66.4	65.8	65.3	64.9	64.5	64.2	64.1	63.9	63.7	63.5	63.4	63.3	63.3	63.2	63.1	63.1	63.1	63.0	63.0
64	68.7	67.9	67.4	66.9	66.4	65.9	65.5	65.2	65.1	64.9	64.7	64.5	64.4	64.3	64.3	64.2	64.1	64.1	64.1	64.0	64.0
65	69.7	69.0	68.5	67.9	67.4	66.9	66.5	66.3	66.1	65.9	65.7	65.5	65.4	65.3	65.3	65.2	65.1	65.1	65.1	65.0	65.0
66	70.8	70.1	69.5	69.0	68.5	68.0	67.6	67.3	67.1	66.9	66.7	66.5	66.4	66.3	66.3	66.2	66.1	66.1	66.1	66.0	66.0
67	71.9	71.1	70.6	70.0	69.5	69.0	68.6	68.3	68.2	68.0	67.7	67.5	67.4	67.3	67.3	67.2	67.1	67.1	67.1	67.0	67.0
68	73.0	72.2	71.7	71.1	70.5	70.0	69.6	69.3	69.2	69.0	68.8	68.6	68.4	68.3	68.3	68.2	68.1	68.1	68.1	68.0	68.0
69	74.0	73.2	72.7	72.1	71.6	71.1	70.6	70.3	70.2	70.0	69.8	69.6	69.4	69.3	69.3	69.2	69.1	69.1	69.1	69.0	69.0
70			74.3	73.8	73.1	72.6	72.1	71.6	71.4	71.2	71.0	70.8	70.6	70.4	70.3	70.2	70.1	70.1	70.1	70.0	70.0
71				74.8	74.2	73.6	73.1	72.7	72.4	72.2	72.0	71.8	71.6	71.4	71.3	71.2	71.1	71.1	71.1	71.0	71.0
72					74.7	74.2	73.7	73.4	73.3	73.0	72.8	72.6	72.4	72.4	72.3	72.2	72.1	72.1	72.1	72.0	72.0
73							74.7	74.4	74.3	74.0	73.8	73.6	73.4	73.4	73.3	73.2	73.1	73.1	73.1	73.0	73.0
74											74.8	74.6	74.4	74.4	74.3	74.2	74.1	74.1	74.1	74.0	74.0

FIG. 87.

1. Technique

The foregoing tables (Figs. 77-87) are used in conjunction with Greulich-Pyle standards (see pp. 74-79).

2. Measurements

See Figures 77-87.

In each table, the skeletal ages are given across the top, with the corresponding percentage of mature height directly below its skeletal age derived from the standards of Greulich and Pyle. Mature heights may be compiled from these percentages by dividing the child's height by the percentage which corresponds to his skeletal age, or predicted height may be read directly from the tables. It is important to use the correct table for the child's sex and to select the table suitable for his rate of maturing. When within one year of a child's chronologic age, use Figures 77 and 78 for boys and Figures 82 and 83 for girls; when accelerated a year or more, use Figures 79 and 80, or 84 and 85; and when retarded a year or more, use Figure 81 or Figures 86 and 87.

3. Source of Material

These tables have been constructed from data on 192 normal children (103 girls and 89 boys) who were measured and radiographed every 6 months from 8 years through 18 years, or until all epiphyses of the hand were closed. The tables were then validated by applying them to a different group of 46 children (23 boys and 23 girls).

GROWTH ESTIMATE FOR RADIUS AND ULNA*

The table below is of value for estimating the degree of acceleration or retardation of the growth of these bones at any age prior to the 25th month.

AGE (MO.)	NO. OF CASES	AVERAGE LENGTH (MM.)	RANGE		AVERAGE INCREASE (MM.)	AVERAGE GROWTH PER MONTH (MM. CALCULATED)
			Shortest (Mm.)	Longest (Mm.)		
White Male						
RADIUS						
3	100	65.90	58	73	.....	.....
6	100	73.10	66	81	7.20	2.40
9	100	80.01	73	90	6.91	2.30
12	100	85.72	75.5	95	5.71	1.90
18	100	94.84	84	107	9.02	1.50
24	100	102.37	95	115.5	7.63	1.27
ULNA						
3	100	73.55	65	82.5	.....	.....
6	100	81.03	73	90.5	7.48	2.49
9	100	88.20	80	98	7.17	2.39
12	100	94.84	85	104.5	6.60	2.21
18	100	104.99	93	115	10.15	1.69
24	100	112.64	102	125	7.65	1.28
White Female						
RADIUS						
3	100	62.85	54	70	.....	.....
6	100	69.73	60	78	6.88	2.29
9	100	76.18	66.5	84	6.46	2.15
12	100	81.73	71	91	5.55	1.85
18	100	91.70	82	103	9.97	1.66
24	100	99.44	88	112	7.74	1.29
ULNA						
3	100	70.58	61	80	.....	.....
6	100	77.67	69	87	7.09	2.36
9	100	84.70	75	93	7.03	2.34
12	100	90.73	80	102	6.03	2.01
18	100	101.62	90	115	10.89	1.81
24	100	109.79	97	124	8.17	1.36

FIG. 88.—(From Ghantus, Table I.)

*Ghantus, M. K.: Am. J. Roentgenol. 65:784, 1951.

1. *Technique*

    a) Central ray: Perpendicular to the plane of the film.

    b) Position: Anteroposterior projection of the forearm with the part pronated and firmly applied on the cassette.

    c) Target-film distance: 36 inches.

2. *Measurements*

See Figure 88.

    Films were taken only within 5 days before or after each specified age. The distance from the proximal end to the distal end of the shadow of the shaft was determined to the nearest 0.5 mm.

3. *Source of Material*

Material of the Brush Foundation, Western Reserve University, was used. Serial roentgenograms of healthy white children only were used. One hundred films were studied for each age group in each set—1,200 films and 2,400 measurements in all.

A. Metacarpal Sign*

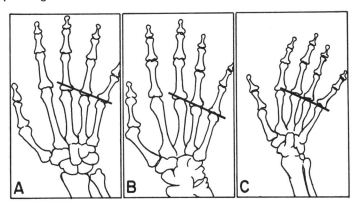

FIG. 89.—The metacarpal sign: *A*, negative; *B*, borderline; *C*, positive.

B. The Carpal Sign†

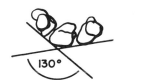

NORMAL   **TURNER'S SYNDROME**

FIG. 90.—From Keats, T. E., and Burns, T. W.: Radiol. Clin. North America 2:297, 1964.

C. Phalangeal Sign‡

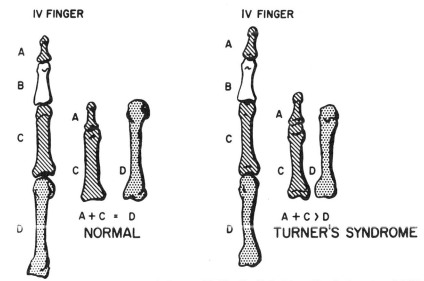

FIG. 91.—From Keats, T. E., and Burns, T. W.: Radiol. Clin. North America 2:297, 1964.

*Archibald, R. M., *et al.*: J. Clin. Endocrinol. 19:1312, 1959.

†Kosowicz, J.: J. Clin. Endocrinol. 22:949, 1962.

‡Kosowicz, J.: Am. J. Roentgenol. 93:354, 1965.

HAND MEASUREMENTS FOR DETECTION OF GONADAL DYSGENESIS

1. *Technique*
    a) Central ray: Perpendicular to plane of film centered over palm.
    b) Projection: Posteroanterior.
    c) Target-film distance: Immaterial.

2. *Measurements*
    A. Metacarpal sign (Fig. 89): A line drawn tangentially to the distal end of the heads of the 5th and 4th metacarpals extends distally to the head of the 3d metacarpal. A positive sign is present when the line passes through the head of the 3d metacarpal. When the line is tangential to the head of the third metacarpal, the sign is considered borderline. A positive metacarpal sign, while not diagnostic in itself, is an accessory sign of gonadal dysgenesis to be correlated with other radiographic and clinical findings. It has no significance when detectable in more than one generation.

    B. The carpal sign (Fig. 90): Two tangents are drawn, the first touching the proximal contour of the navicular and lunate bones and the second touching the triangular and lunate bones. In normal subjects, a value of 131.5° is obtained. In patients with gonadal dysgenesis, the carpal angle is 117° or less.

    C. The phalangeal sign (Fig. 91): Comparison of the length of the 4th metacarpal with the total length of the distal plus proximal phalanges of the 4th finger in normal subjects indicates equal dimensions of these bones; the differences do not exceed 2 mm. In some cases of gonadal aplasia, the total height of the distal and proximal phalanges exceeds by 3 mm. or more the height of the 4th metacarpal.

3. *Source of Material*

    The metacarpal sign is based on a study of 2,594 unselected patients. The carpal and phalangeal signs of Kosowicz are based on measurements of 466 normal subjects.

C. The Spine

MEASUREMENT OF ATLAS-ODONTOID DISTANCE

This measurement is useful in the diagnosis of minimum atlantoaxial subluxation.

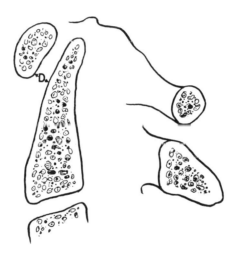

FIG. 92.

Normal range:

1. Adult (average normal in mm.):*

    Female: $D_F = 1.238 - (0.0074 \times \text{Age in years}) \pm 0.90$ mm.
    Between ages of 20 and 80 years.

    Male: $D_M = 2.052 - (0.0192 \times \text{Age in years}) \pm 1.00$ mm.
    Between ages of 30 and 80 years

2. Children (average normal in mm.):†

    $D = 2.0$; 99% of patients will be between 1 mm. and 4 mm.
    Maximum distance found in a normal patient was 5 mm

---

*Hinck, V. C., and Hopkins, C. E.: Am. J. Roentgenol. 84:945, 1960.

†Locke, G. R.; Gardner, J. I.; and Van Epps, E. F.: Am. J. Roentgenol. 97:135, 1966.

MEASUREMENT OF ATLAS-ODONTOID DISTANCE

1. *Technique*

  a) Central ray: Perpendicular to plane of film centered at level of thyroid cartilage.

  b) Position: Lateral. Patient sitting with head in "neutral" position.

  c) Target-film distance: 72 inches.

2. *Measurements*

  See Figure 92.

  Measurement is made between the posteroinferior margin of the anterior arch of the atlas and the anterior surface of the odontoid process.

  There is a significant difference between measurements in extension and in neutral position, but there is a negligible difference between flexion and neutral position.* Ninety-five per cent of normal adults will have an atlas-odontoid distance in flexion between 0.3 and 1.8 mm., in neutral position between 0.4 mm. and 2.0 mm., and in extension between 0.3 and 2.2 mm.* Neutral position is recommended for children.

3. *Source of Material*

  Hinck studied 25 adult males (30-80 years) and 25 adult females (20-80 years).

  Locke studied 200 children whose ages ranged from 3 to 15 years. Lateral roentgenograms were made in neutral, flexion and extension positions at target-film distances of 72 inches (patient sitting) and 40 inches (patient supine). Neutral position is recommended because flexion at both 72- and 40-inch distances tends to increase the atlas-odontoid distance, as does extension at a 40-inch distance.

---

*Hinck, V. C., and Hopkins, C. E.: Am. J. Roentgenol. 84:945, 1960.

MEASUREMENT OF THE SAGITTAL DIAMETER
OF THE CERVICAL SPINAL CANAL IN INFANTS*

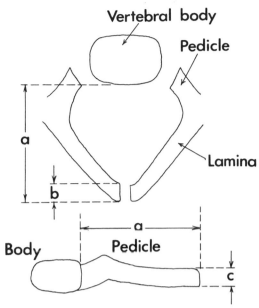

FIG. 93.—Cervical spinal canal in infants: a, distance from posterior border of vertebral body to tip of the spinous process; b, thickness (in dissected specimen) of the spinous process; c, height (on lateral radiograph) of the spinous process. At this age $b - c$. (Redrawn from Naik, Fig. 1.)

1. Technique

a) Central ray: Projected to the 7th cervical vertebra.
b) Position: True lateral.
c) Target-film distance: 90 cm.

2. Measurements

See Figure 93.
The sagittal diameter can be determined by measuring from the posterior border of the vertebral body to the posterior end of the laminae (distance a) and subtracting the height (c) of the laminae. Sagittal diameter of the spinal canal = $a-c$.

Sagittal Diameter of Spinal Canal

Vertebral Level	Mean Diameter in mm.
C_2	12.5
C_3	11.5
C_4	11.5
C_5	12.2
C_6	12.6
C_7	12.1

Standard deviation is 0.7 mm. (From Naik, Table 1.)

3. Source of Material

Twenty-five normal spines in infants under 12 months of age were studied post mortem.

*Naik, D. R.: Clin. Radiol. 21:323, 1970 (By kind permission of the honorary editor of Clinical Radiology.)

MEASUREMENT OF THE SAGITTAL DIAMETER OF THE
CERVICAL SPINAL CANAL IN CHILDREN*

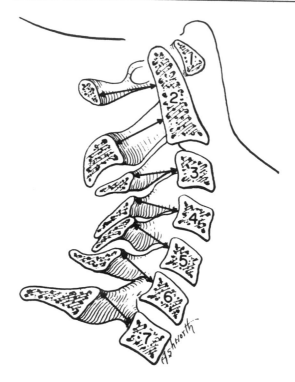

FIG. 94.—(From Hinck, Hopkins, and Savara, Fig. 1.)

1. *Technique*

   a) Central ray: Projected through the 4th cervical vertebra.

   b) Position: True lateral. Patient seated with the head in neutral position.

   c) Target-film distance: 5 feet distance from target to midsagittal plane of spine. Distance from midplane to cassette varied up to 2.5 cm.

2. *Measurements*

   See Figures 94-96.

   The sagittal diameter was measured from the middle of the posterior surface of the ventral body to the nearest point on the ventral line of the cortex seen at the junction of spinous processes and laminae *(arrows)*.

*Hinck, V. C.; Hopkins, C. E.; and Savara, B. S.: Radiology 79:97, 1962.

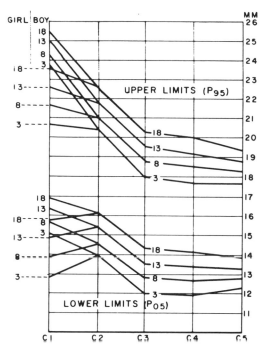

FIG. 95.—(From Hinck, Hopkins, and Savara, Fig. 3.)

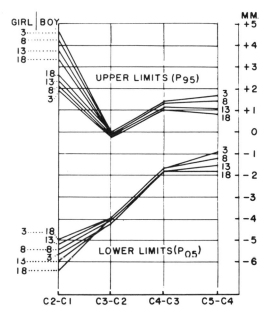

FIG. 96.—(From Hinck, Hopkins, and Savara, Fig. 4.)

Ninety per cent tolerance limits for sagittal diameters of C1-C5 in boys and girls from 3 to 18 years of age.

Ninety per cent tolerance limits for sagittal diameter differences between adjacent vertebrae, C1-C5, in boys and girls from 3 to 18 years of age.

3. Source of Material

Measurements were made on 333 films, using the Bolton-Broadbent cephalometer, on 48 white children aged 3-18 years, at annual intervals.

MEASUREMENT OF THE SAGITTAL DIAMETER OF THE CERVICAL SPINAL CANAL IN ADULTS

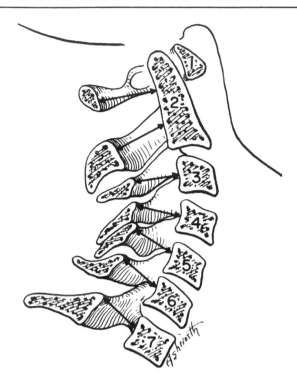

FIG. 97.—(From Hinck, Hopkins, and Savara, Fig. 1.)*

1. *Technique*

   a) Central ray: Projected through the 4th cervical vertebra.
   b) Position: True lateral. Patient seated with the head in neutral position.
   c) Target-film distance: 73.8 inches. Target-table top distance was 72 inches, and table top to film in Bucky tray was 1.8 inches.

2. *Measurements*

   See Figure 97.
   The sagittal diameter was measured from the middle of the posterior surface of the ventral body to the nearest point on the ventral line of the cortex seen at the junction of spinous processes and laminae *(arrows)*.

*Hinck, V. C.; Hopkins, C. E.; and Savara, B. S.: Radiology 79:97, 1962.

MEASUREMENT OF THE SAGITTAL DIAMETER
OF THE CERVICAL SPINAL CORD IN ADULTS*

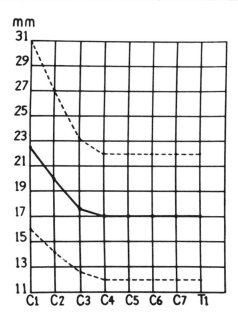

(From Wolf, Khilnani, and Malis,
Fig. 3.*)

Curves for average, maximal, and
minimal sagittal measurements of cervical spinal canal in adults.* Plotted
values are uncorrected measurements
from lateral neck films taken at 72
inch target-table top distance. True
measurements are 1.5 mm. less than
those shown.

3. *Source of Material*

Measurements were made on 200 adults with no known neurological disturbances
and showing no obvious bone or joint changes on the films.

---

*Wolf, B. S.; Khilnani, M.; and Malis, L.: J. Mt. Sinai Hosp., New York 23:283, 1956.

MEASUREMENT OF THE SAGITTAL DIAMETER OF THE CERVICAL* AND THORACIC† SPINAL CORD IN ADULTS

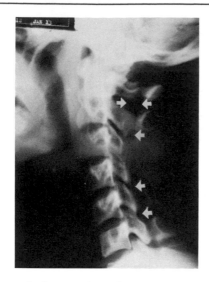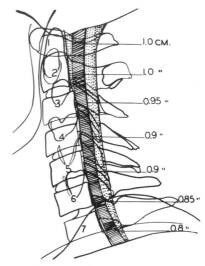

FIG. 98.—*Left*, normal myelogram of cervical area. Posterior limits of cord indicated by arrows. *Right*, diagrammatic tracing showing average normal measurements for cervical levels. (From Lowman and Finkelstein, Fig. 2.)

VERTEBRAL LEVELS	MEASUREMENT		
	MIN. (MM.)	AV. (MM.)	MAX. (MM.)
C_1	8.0	10.0	11.0
C_2	8.0	10.0	11.0
C_3	7.5	9.5	10.0
C_4	7.5	9.0	10.0
C_5	7.5	9.0	9.0
C_6	7.5	8.5	9.0
C_7	7.5	8.0	9.0
D_3		6.0	
D_4	5.6	6.2	7.3
D_5	3.7	6.1	7.2
D_6	3.7	6.1	7.8
D_7	5.3	6.3	7.9
D_8	3.4	6.3	7.8
D_9	3.7	6.2	8.0
D_{10}	6.0	6.5	7.0
D_{11}	4.5	6.9	10.5
D_{12}	3.8	7.4	9.3

1. *Technique*

   a) Central ray: Cervical—Projected through the 4th cervical vertebra.
      Thoracic—Lateral thoracic myelogram.
   b) Position: Cervical—Erect true lateral. Caldwell position with the film alongside the shoulder.
      Thoracic—Lateral thoracic myelogram.
   c) Target-film distance: Cervical—72 inches.
      Thoracic—Variable with myelogram.

---

*Lowman, R. M., and Finkelstein, A.: Radiology 39:700, 1942.

†Jirout, J.: Fortschr. Geb. Röntgenstrahlen 104:89, 1966.

2. *Measurements*

See Figure 98. Diameters are given at vertebral body level.

3. *Source of Material*

   a) Cervical: 80 normal encephalograms in which the upper cervical area was included on the lateral film of the skull and on 30 normal air myelograms.
   b) Thoracic: Measured on all myelograms for lumbar disc pathology, 1953-1965, at Neurologische Klinik, Prague.

MEASUREMENT OF THE WIDTH
OF THE CERVICAL SPINAL CORD IN ADULTS*

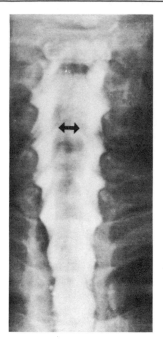

FIG. 99.—Normal cervical myelogram demonstrating method of measurement. (From Porter, Fig. 1.)

1. *Technique*

a) Central ray: Centered over midportion of the cervical spine.

b) Position: Posteroanterior.

c) Target-film distance: Measurements from spot films were made at fluoroscopy, and the anode-to-spine and the spine-to-film distance varied to some extent. The average target-film distance was 33 inches.

2. *Measurements*

See Figure 99.

Measurements were made at the level of the 4th and 6th cervical vertebrae when possible. The distance between the "inner" shadow of the true cord was measured rather than the entire central shadow, which includes the nerve roots.

$$
\begin{aligned}
\text{Average width} &= 1.4 \text{ cm.} \\
\text{Minimum width} &= 1.0 \text{ cm.} \\
\text{Maximum width} &= 1.7 \text{ cm.}
\end{aligned}
$$

3. *Source of Material*

The measurements were based on cervical myelograms of 63 patients who showed either ruptured intervertebral disks or no pathology at operation.

*Porter, E. C.: Am. J. Roentgenol. 76:270, 1956.

MEASUREMENT OF THE SAGITTAL DIAMETER OF THE LUMBAR SPINAL CANAL IN CHILDREN AND ADULTS*

1. *Technique*

   a) Central ray: Perpendicular to plane of film centered at level of 3d lumbar vertebral body.

   b) Position: Lateral lumbar spine.

   c) Target-film distance: 40 inches.

2. *Measurements*

   The sagittal diameter of the spinal canal is measured at the level of each lumbar vertebra. The sagittal diameter is the shortest midline perpendicular distance from the posterior surface of the vertebral body to the inner surface of the neural arch.

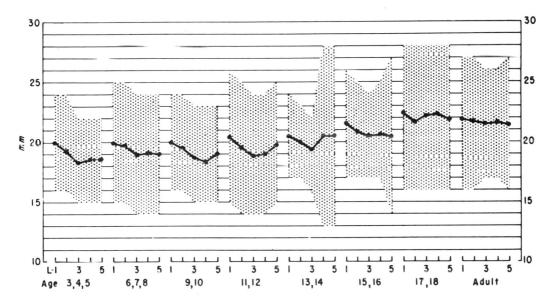

   Age group means and 90 per cent tolerance limits for the sagittal diameter of the spinal canal of each lumbar vertebra, male and female combined. (From Hinck, Hopkins, and Clark, Fig. 1.)

*Hinck, V. C.; Hopkins, C. E.; and Clark, W. M.: Radiology 85:929, 1965.

MEASUREMENT OF THE SAGITTAL DIAMETER OF THE LUMBAR SPINAL CANAL IN CHILDREN AND ADULTS

AGE-GROUP MEANS AND STANDARD DEVIATIONS, BY SEX (MM.)*

Vertebra	N†	Male Mean	S.D.	N†	Female Mean	S.D.	N†	Male Mean	S.D.	N†	Female Mean	S.D.
		Age 3, 4, 5 years						Age 6, 7, 8 years				
L1	15	20.3	1.8	9	19.8	1.2	14	20.3	1.9	10	19.3	2.6
2	15	19.6	1.2	9	18.9	1.4	15	19.9	1.7	9	19.5	1.6
3	15	18.4	1.4	9	18.1	1.4	15	19.1	1.8	10	18.4	1.6
4	15	18.8	1.1	9	18.0	1.5	15	19.0	1.7	10	19.1	1.8
5	14	19.0	1.6	9	17.5	1.4	15	19.0	2.4	10	19.1	2.3
		Age 9, 10 years						Age 11, 12 years				
L1	8	20.1	1.0	4	19.8	1.9	5	22.6	2.0	11	19.6	1.1
2	8	19.6	1.0	5	19.6	1.7	5	21.2	2.7	11	18.9	1.7
3	8	18.8	1.6	5	18.9	1.3	5	19.9	2.9	11	18.4	1.4
4	8	18.6	1.7	5	18.6	1.2	5	18.8	3.0	11	19.1	1.7
5	8	19.1	1.9	5	18.9	1.1	5	19.7	2.7	11	19.8	2.4
		Age 13, 14 years						Age 15, 16 years				
L1	14	20.5	1.5	10	20.8	1.4	10	21.6	2.2	18	21.6	2.2
2	14	19.7	1.4	10	20.1	0.9	11	20.8	2.1	18	20.9	1.8
3	14	18.9	1.7	10	20.0	1.3	11	20.5	1.6	18	20.7	1.6
4	14	20.4	4.1	10	20.2	2.5	11	20.0	1.7	18	21.0	2.1
5	14	20.8	4.2	10	20.1	3.2	10	20.1	2.9	18	20.8	3.4
		Age 17, 18 years						Adult				
L1	11	23.9	1.9	17	21.7	1.7	22	22.2	3.1	25	21.3	2.3
2	11	22.4	2.3	17	21.3	1.9	23	22.3	2.7	26	21.2	2.1
3	12	22.6	2.3	18	22.0	3.1	23	21.7	2.6	26	21.3	2.1
4	12	22.9	2.8	18	21.9	2.6	23	21.8	2.4	26	21.3	1.9
5	12	22.6	3.4	18	21.4	2.2	21	22.6	2.7	25	20.4	2.4

*Hinck, V. C.; Hopkins, C. E.; and Clark, W. M.: Radiology 85:929, 1965.

†N = Number of subjects.

(From Hinck, Hopkins, and Clark, Table I.)

3. Source of Material

Films were selected on the basis of readability, and an attempt was made to eliminate subjects who showed significant anomalies and other problems likely to influence growth and development. The number of subjects in each group is shown in the above table.

1. *Technique*

    a) Central ray: Perpendicular to plane of film centered over midportion of segment of spine being examined.

    b) Position: Anteroposterior.

    c) Target-film distance: 40 inches.

2. *Measurements*

    See Figures 100–108.

    Interpediculate distance is the shortest distance between the medial surfaces of the pedicles of a given vertebra.

    Figures 101-108 from Hinck *et al.** show a shaded area for each graph which is the 90% tolerance range. These tolerance ranges are the high and low limits within which the central 90% of "normals" may be expected to fall.

    Figure 100 from Schwarz† shows the "extreme upper limits" for the normal spinal canal in newborns to adults.

3. *Source of Material*

    Hinck used 474 radiographs, including 353 children (under age 19 years) and 121 adults. Radiographs were selected from the files of the University of Oregon Medical School, and an attempt was made to eliminate subjects with significant anomalies and problems likely to influence growth and development.

    Schwarz used radiographs of 200 patients.

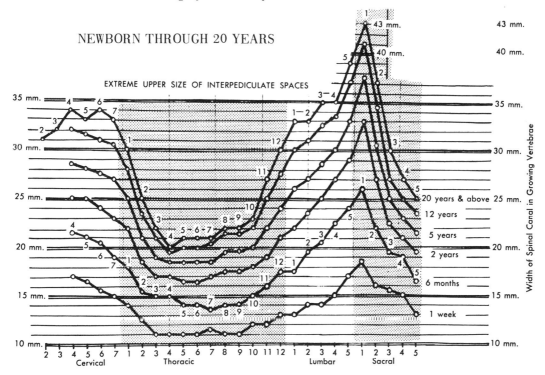

FIG. 100.—All curves delineate the maximum measurement observed for a given vertebra at the age designated. (Adapted from Schwarz†.)

---

*Hinck, V. C., *et al.*: Am. J. Roentgenol. 97:141, 1966.

†Schwarz, G. S.: Am. J. Roentgenol. 76:476, 1956.

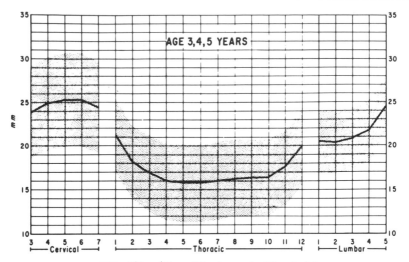

FIG. 101.—(From Hinck *et al.*, Fig. 3,*A.*)

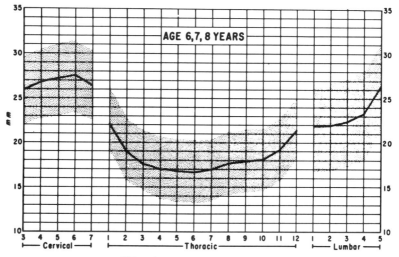

FIG. 102.—(From Hinck *et al.*, Fig. 3,*B.*)

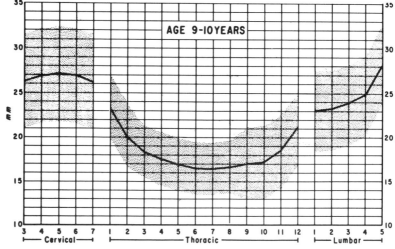

FIG. 103.—(From Hinck *et al.*, Fig. 3,*C.*)

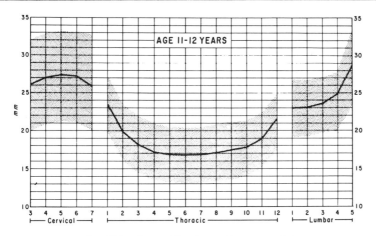

FIG. 104. — (From Hinck *et al.*, Fig. 3,*D*.)

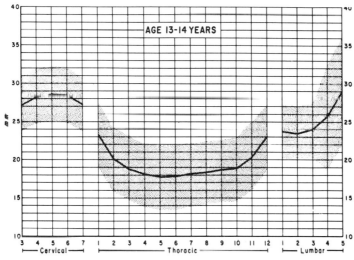

FIG. 105. — (From Hinck *et al.*, Fig. 3,*E*.)

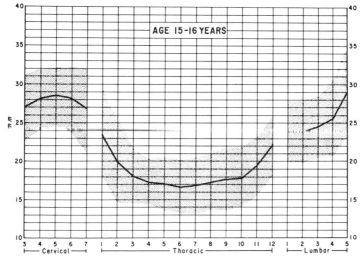

FIG. 106. — (From Hinck *et al.*, Fig. 3,*F*.)

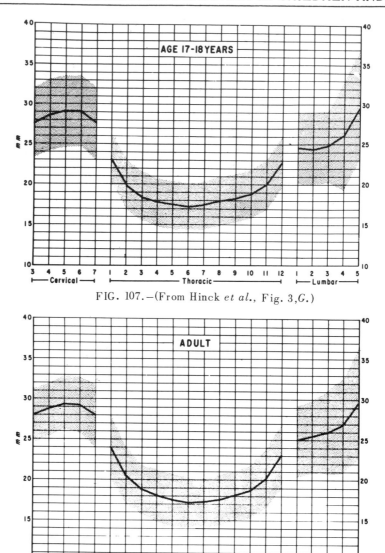

FIG. 107.—(From Hinck *et al.*, Fig. 3,*G*.)

FIG. 108.—(From Hinck *et al.*, Fig. 3,*H*.)

VERTEBRAL BODY AND INTERVERTEBRAL DISC INDEX IN CHILDREN
(12th THORACIC TO 3rd LUMBAR)

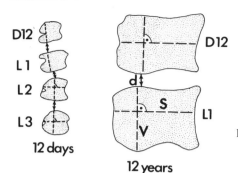

FIG. 109. –(Redrawn from Brandner,* Fig. 1.)

1. *Technique*

   a) Central ray: Projected through 1st lumbar vertebra.
   b) Position: True lateral projection with Bucky table.
   c) Target-film distance: 110 cm. However, indices are independent of target-film distance.

2. *Measurements*

   See Figure 109.

   I_{vb} = Vertebral body index = $\dfrac{v}{s}$ = $\dfrac{\text{Height of vertebral body}}{\text{Sagittal diameter of vertebral body}}$

   Height is the largest vertical measurement of the body.
   Sagittal diameter is the smallest anteroposterior measurement of the body.

   I_d = Intervertebral disc index = $\dfrac{d}{v}$ = $\dfrac{\text{Intervertebral disc thickness}}{\text{Height of vertebral body}}$

   Upper disc and lower vertebral body are compared.

---

*Brandner, M. E.: Am. J. Roentgenol. 110:618, 1970.

VERTEBRAL BODY AND INTERVERTEBRAL DISC INDEX IN CHILDREN
(12th THORACIC TO 3rd LUMBAR)

I_{vb} (v/s) OF VERTEBRAL BODIES[†]

Vertebral Body	Age Group	N	Mean v/s
D12	0-1 month	13	0.81
	2-18 months	26	0.91
	19-36 months	22	0.86
	4-12 years (F)	18	0.86
	4-12 years (M)	35	0.78
	13 years and over (F)	7	0.93
	13 years and over (M)	20	0.84
L1	0-1 month	16	0.87
	2-18 months (F)	11	1.02
	2-18 months (M)	16	0.96
	2-18 months (M & F)	27	0.98
	19-36 months	23	0.89
	4-12 years (F)	20	0.87
	4-12 years (M)	40	0.80
	13 years and over (F)	19	1.03
	13 years and over (M)	27	0.87
L2	0-1 month	10	0.92
	2-18 months	21	1.01
	19-36 months	20	0.91
	4-12 years	49	0.82
	13 years and over (F)	15	1.03
	13 years and over (M)	25	0.88
L3	0-1 month	11	0.95
	2-18 months	17	0.98
	19-36 months	16	0.88
	4-12 years	35	0.79
	13 years and over (F)	11	1.00
	13 years and over (M)	17	0.87

N = number of subjects.
F = female; M = male.

[†]Adapted from Brandner, Table 3.

VERTEBRAL BODY AND INTERVERTEBRAL DISC INDEX IN CHILDREN
(12th THORACIC TO 3rd LUMBAR)

I_d (d/v) OF INTERVERTEBRAL DISC AND VERTEBRAL BODY*

Vertebral Segment	Age Group	N	Mean d/v
D 11/12	0-1 month	12	0.37
	2-18 months	26	0.30
	19-36 months	19	0.25
	4-12 years	49	0.24
	13 years and over	21	0.18
D 12/L1	0-1 month	17	0.35
	2-18 months	27	0.28
	19-36 months	20	0.26
	4-12 years	53	0.25
	13 years and over	37	0.19
L 1/2	0-1 month	15	0.35
	2-18 months	26	0.26
	19-36 months	19	0.27
	4-12 years	44	0.28
	13 years and over	37	0.20
L 2/3	0-1 month	9	0.38
	2-18 months	18	0.28
	19-36 months	15	0.30
	4-12 years	32	0.30
	13 years and over	22	0.21

N = number of subjects.

3. Source of Material

Brandner studied 187 roentgenograms of dorsal and lumbar spines from newborns to adolescents.

---

*Adapted from Brandner, Table 4.

MEASUREMENT OF VERTEBRAL BODY HEIGHT
AND INTERVERTEBRAL DISC WIDTH – DORSAL
AND LUMBAR REGIONS IN FEMALES*

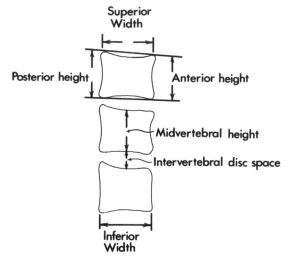

FIG. 110.

1. *Technique*

   a) Central ray: Dorsal spine—Projected through 9th dorsal vertebra.
   Lumbar spine—Projected through 3rd lumbar vertebra.
   b) Position: True lateral. Patient lying on left side.
   c) Target-film distance: 40 inches.

2. *Measurements*

   See Figure 110.

*Hurxthal, L. M.: Am. J. Roentgenol. 103:635, 1968.

116

MEASUREMENT OF VERTEBRAL BODY HEIGHT
AND INTERVERTEBRAL DISC WIDTH – DORSAL
AND LUMBAR REGIONS IN FEMALES

Inter-vertebral Disc or Vertebra Level	Mean Inter-vertebral Disc Space (mm.)	Mean Height of Anterior Vertebral Border (mm.)	Mean Height of Posterior Vertebral Border (mm.)	Mean Midline Height of Vertebra (mm.)	Mean Width of Superior Border of Vertebra (mm.)	Mean Width of Inferior Border of Vertebra (mm.)	Range in Disc Space (mm.)
L5-4 + L5	11.0	35.4	32.2	31.0	37.8	39.6	8-14
L4-3 + L4	10.2	35.1	33.7	28.0	39.0	38.3	7-17
L3-2 + L3	10.2	34.7	34.3	34.0	37.0	37.6	6-16
L2-1 + L2	7.9	32.9	33.7	29.0	34.9	36.5	3-10
L1-D12 + L1	6.9	31.7	32.4	31.0	35.8	33.3	5-12
D12-11 + D12	6.4	28.7	28.5	31.5	35.5	34.0	4-12
D11-10 + D11	4.7	26.7	27.1	28.5	35.2	35.2	4-8
D10-9 + D10	4.4	26.5	26.0	25.0	35.0	35.1	4-7
D9-8 + D9	4.4	24.8	24.9	25.0	33.8	33.8	4-5
D8-7 + D8	4.4	23.3	24.0	23.0	31.1	31.7	4-1
D7-6 + D7	4.0	23.5	23.7	22.0	29.6	31.4	3-8
Totals in mm. (to nearest integral)							
Younger group	75	323	321	308	386	388	3-17
Older group	84	321	337	316	386	395	3-14

Mean age

Younger group   22 years (15-30)

Older group   62 years (47-75)

(From Hurxthal, Table 1.)

3. *Source of Material*

Hurxthal measured 220 vertebrae on 20 lateral roentgenograms of dorsal and lumbar spines selected from ambulatory women in good health. Ten subjects were between ages 15 years and 30 years and 10 subjects were between ages 47 years and 75 years.

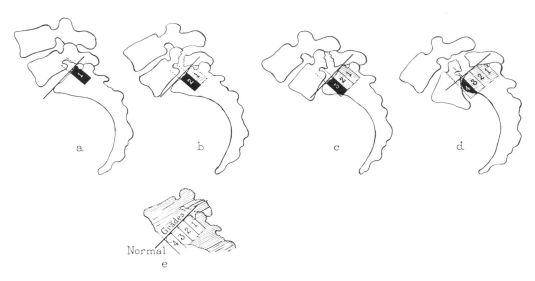

FIG. 111.—Meyerding's method of classifying the degree of spondylolisthesis. (From Meyerding, H. W.: Surg., Gynec. & Obst. 54:374 [Fig. 3], 1932.)

1. *Technique*

   a) Central ray: Centered over lumbosacral junction perpendicular to plane of film.
   b) Position: True lateral. Upright and horizontal positions may be necessary to demonstrate spondylolisthesis.
   c) Target-film distance: Immaterial. Distance of at least 36 inches desirable.

2. *Measurements*

   a) Meyerding's classification scheme (Fig. 111) is based, not on actual measurements, but on the position of the posterior aspect of the body of the 5th lumbar vertebra in relation to the superior surface of the 1st sacral segment, which is divided into quarters.
   b) Garland and Thomas' vertical line (Fig. 112) is drawn perpendicular to the upper surface of the 1st sacral body at its anterior superior margin. In all normal individuals the anterior inferior margin of the 5th lumbar body lay from 1 to 8 mm. behind this line.

3. *Source of Material*

   a) Meyerding's classification is based on observations made on 207 cases of spondylolisthesis between 1918 and 1931.
   b) Garland and Thomas' data is based on a study of 170 cases. Twenty of these had neural arch defects; and of the 20, 8 showed spondylolisthesis, according to his criteria.

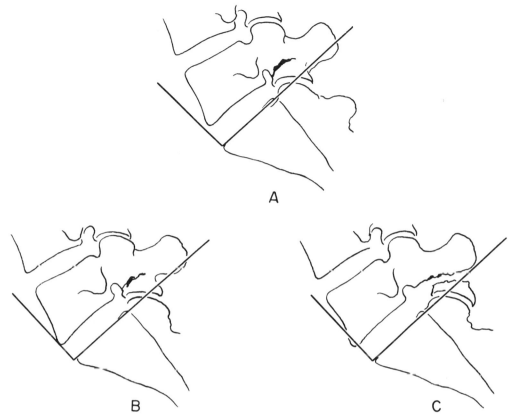

FIG. 112.—Diagram illustrating use of the right-angle test line for diagnosis of anterior spondylolisthesis. *A*, neural arch defects without slip. Note that the anterior margin of the 5th lumbar body lies about 3mm. behind the test line. *B*, neural arch defects without definite slip. The body of the 5th lumbar vertebra does touch the test line, but its posterior edge is not significantly out of line and none of the other findings of olisthesis are present. Occasionally, defects of this type can be shown to slip slightly in the erect position. *C*, spondylolisthesis, partial grade 1. The anterior margin of the 5th lumbar body crosses the test line. (Adapted from Garland, L. H., and Thomas, S. F.: Am. J. Roentgenol. 55:275, 1946.)

MEASUREMENT OF THE LUMBOSACRAL ANGLE*

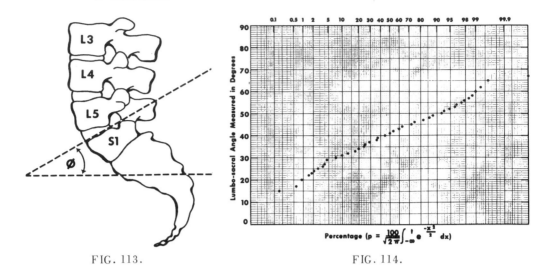

FIG. 113.   FIG. 114.

1. *Technique*

    a) Central ray: Perpendicular to plane of film. Upright spot films of L5-S1 inter-
       vertebral space centered 1 inch below iliac crest.
    b) Position: True lateral with patient standing.
    c) Target-film distance: 40 inches.

2. *Measurements*

    See Figure 113.
    Line of inclination is the plane of the 1st sacral surface.
      Line of horizontal is drawn parallel to the bottom margin of the film.
    Lumbosacral angle is ϕ.
      Mean lumbosacral angle = 41.1°. S. D. = 7.7°. Ninety-five percent of all
    values will lie between 25.7° and 56.5°.
      Values in the study approximated a normal distribution.

    See Figure 114.
      By using this graph it is possible to find the percentage of individuals above
    or below a given value. For example, an angle of 50° shows 92% of individuals less
    than that angle and 8% greater.
      When supine and standing views are compared, there is usually an increase in
    the lumbosacral angle of 8° to 12° in the standing position.

3. *Source of Material*

    Hellems and Keats used 319 normal males ranging in age from 17 to 58 years who had
    lumbosacral spine films made as part of a routine pre-employment examination.

---

*Hellems, H. K., and Keats, T. E.: Am. J. Roentgenol. 113:642, 1971.

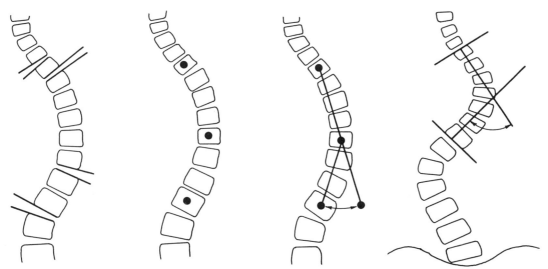

FIG. 115.—Method of Ferguson. (Redrawn from Kittleson and Lim, Figs. 3 and 4.)

FIG. 116.—Method of Cobb. (Redrawn from Kittleson and Lim, Figs. 3 and 4.)

FIG. 117.—(From Meschan, I.: *Roentgen Signs in Clinical Diagnosis* [Philadelphia: W. B. Saunders Company, 1956], p. 453, Figs. 14-24 and 14-25.)

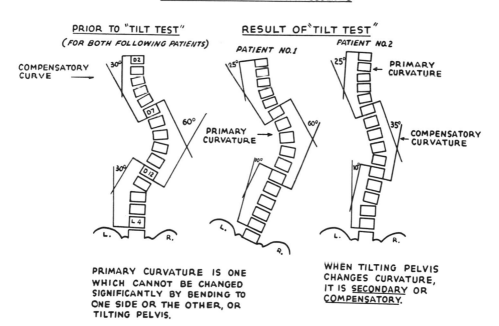

DETERMINATION OF PRIMARY AND SECONDARY
CURVATURES IN DORSAL SCOLIOSIS

PRIOR TO "TILT TEST"
(FOR BOTH FOLLOWING PATIENTS)

RESULT OF "TILT TEST"

PATIENT NO.1

PATIENT NO.2

COMPENSATORY CURVE

PRIMARY CURVATURE

COMPENSATORY CURVATURE

PRIMARY CURVATURE

PRIMARY CURVATURE IS ONE WHICH CANNOT BE CHANGED SIGNIFICANTLY BY BENDING TO ONE SIDE OR THE OTHER, OR TILTING PELVIS.

WHEN TILTING PELVIS CHANGES CURVATURE, IT IS SECONDARY OR COMPENSATORY.

*Ferguson, A. B.: *Roentgen Diagnosis of Extremities and Spine* (New York: Paul B. Hoeber, Inc., 1949).

†Cobb, J. R.: Am. Acad. Orthop. Surg. 5:261-275, 1948.

MEASUREMENT OF SCOLIOSIS

1. *Technique*

   a) Central ray: Perpendicular to plane of film centered over dorsolumbar junction.
   b) Position: Anteroposterior.
   c) Target-film distance: Immaterial.

2. *Measurements*

See Figures 115 and 116. The secondary curvatures function to bring the head erect over the pelvis and keep the body in balance in the erect posture. When the primary curve is not definitely identified, examination is made with the patient seated with the pelvis elevated 4 inches (by sandbag or otherwise) on the side of the convexity of the lumbar curve. No support is allowed the patient. In this posture the muscles at the convex aspect of the lumbar curve cause marked straightening throughout that curve if it is compensatory, but little or no straightening (except possibly at the end of the curve) if it is primary.

The Ferguson and Cobb methods are two systems for measurement of scoliosis. The Scoliosis Research Society has selected the Cobb system as the standard method of measurement.* The Ferguson method should be used for curves under 50°. The Cobb method should be used for curves over 50°.

a) Method of Ferguson (see Fig. 115):
   1. Locate the End Vertebrae—the vertebra at each end of a curve which is the least rotated and lies between the two curves.
   2. Locate the Apex Vertebra—the most rotated vertebra at the peak of the curve.
   3. In each of these three vertebrae, the *center* of the *outline* of the *body* is marked with a dot.
   4. Lines are drawn from the apex to each end vertebra. The angle of the curve is the divergence of these two lines from 180°.

b) Method of Cobb (see Fig. 116):
   1. Locate the Top Vertebra of the curve. It is the highest one whose superior surface tilts to the side of the concavity of the curve to be measured.
   2. Locate the Bottom Vertebra. It is the lowest one whose inferior surface tilts to the side of the concavity of the curve to be measured.
   3. Erect intersecting perpendiculars from the superior surface of the top and the inferior surface of the bottom vertebrae of the curve. The selection of the end vertebrae and the top and bottom vertebrae is aided by studying the disc spaces. All of the vertebrae in a given curve will show widening of the disc space on the convex side of the curve.
   4. The angle formed by these perpendiculars is the angle of the curve.

3. *Source of Material*

Original observations from the clinical work of Ferguson and from Cobb.

---

*Kittleson, A. C., and Lim, L. W.: Am. J. Roentgenol. 108:775, 1970.

D. The Upper Extremity

AXIAL RELATIONSHIPS OF THE SHOULDER* AND MEASUREMENT OF THE JOINT SPACE†

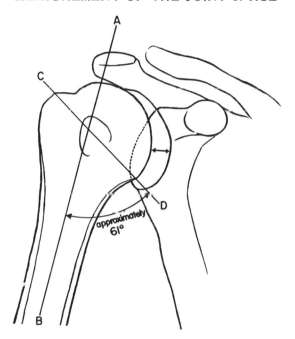

FIG. 118.

Axial Angle

Average for adult females, 62°.
Average for adult males, 60°.

Width of the Joint Space

Adults: 0-6 mm., depending on the degree of rotation of the humerus. More than
6 mm. is significant and is particularly useful in the diagnosis of dislocation of the humeral head.

*Keats, T. E., *et al.*: Radiology 87:904, 1966.

†Arndt, J. H., and Sears, A. D.: Am. J. Roentgenol. 94:638, 1965.

AXIAL RELATIONSHIPS OF THE SHOULDER AND MEASUREMENT OF THE JOINT SPACE

1. *Technique*

   a) Central ray: Perpendicular to the plane of the film centered over the shoulder.

   b) Position: Anteroposterior: external rotation (anatomic position) for axial angle; internal or external rotation for joint space.

   c) Target-film distance: 36-40 inches for joint space. Immaterial for axial angle.

2. *Measurements*

   See Figure 118.

   a) Axial angle:

   AB: Axis of the shaft is drawn between 2 points, each measured to lie in the midline of the diaphysis.

   CD: Axis of the head is drawn between the apex of the greater tuberosity to the junction of the shaft with the distal extremity of the articular surface of the head (the point where the medial cortex changes from a band to a line).

   b) The joint space: Measured between the anterior rim of the glenoid fossa and the medial aspect of the humeral head.

3. *Source of Material*

   Data on the axial angle were derived from a study of 50 normal subjects, equally divided between males and females ranging in age from 17 to 72 years.

   Measurements of the joint space were based on a study of 100 normal shoulders.

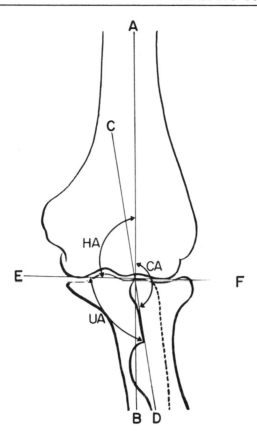

FIG. 119.

MALES

Angle	Min.	Max.	Av.
CA	154°	178°	169°
HA	77°	95°	85°
UA	74°	99°	84°

FEMALES

Angle	Min.	Max.	Av.
CA	158°	178°	167°
HA	72°	91°	83°
UA	72°	93°	84°

*Keats, T. E., *et al.*: Radiology 87:904, 1966.

MEASUREMENT OF THE AXIAL ANGLES AT THE ELBOW

1. *Technique*

    a) Central ray: Perpendicular to plane of film.

    b) Position: Arm fully extended with the two epicondyles perfectly flat with respect to the film.

    c) Target-film distance: Immaterial.

2. *Measurements*

    See Figure 119.

    AB = Line of axis of the shaft of the humerus.

    CD = Line of axis of the shaft of the ulna.

    EF = Transverse line drawn tangentially to the most distal points of the articular surfaces of the trochlea and capitellum.

    CA = The carrying angle formed by the intersection of AB and CD, measured on the radial side.

    HA = The humeral angle formed by the intersection of AB and EF.

    UA = The ulnar angle formed by the intersection of CD and EF.

3. *Source of Material*

    The data have been derived from a study of 50 normal subjects, equally divided between males and females ranging in age from 21 to 66 years.

DETECTION OF DISLOCATION OF THE RADIAL HEAD*

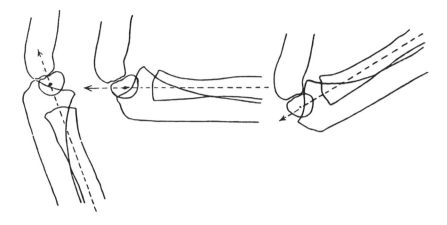

FIG. 120.—(From Storen, Fig. 6.)

1. *Technique*

   a) Central ray: Perpendicular to plane of film centered over joint.
   b) Position: Lateral with elbow flexed.
   c) Target film-distance: Immaterial.

2. *Measurements*

   See Figure 120.

   In the lateral projection, a line extending the radial axis should pass through the center of the capitellum in all stages of flexion of the elbow. This relationship is particularly useful in children, in whom the epiphysial ossification centers have not yet appeared, the gap between the bone ends is wide, and the relationships between the bone ends are difficult to determine.

3. *Source of Material*

   The data are based on the study of approximately 40 patients.

---

*Storen, G.: Acta chir. scandinav. 116:144, 1959.

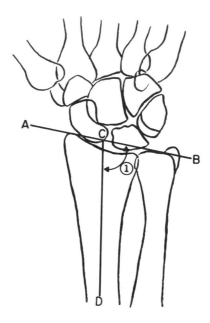

FIG. 121.

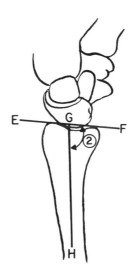

FIG. 122.

	Males	Females	Av.
Angle 1	72°-93°	73°-95°	83°
Angle 2	79°-93°	80°-94°	85.5°

*Keats, T. E., et al.: Radiology 87:904, 1966.

MEASUREMENT OF THE AXIAL ANGLES AT THE WRIST

1. *Technique*

   a) Central ray: Perpendicular to plane of film projected over the navicular bone.
   b) Position: Posteroanterior and lateral.
   c) Target-film distance: Immaterial.

2. *Measurements*

   a) Posteroanterior view (Fig. 121):

   AB = Line drawn tangentially from the distal tip of the radial styloid
      process through the base of the ulnar styloid process.
   CD = Line drawn along the midshaft of the radius.
   Angle *1* = The angle of intersection of AB and CD measured on the ulnar
      side.

   b) Lateral view (Fig. 122):

   EF = Line drawn tangentially across the most distal points of the articular
      surface of the radius.
   GH = Line drawn through the midshaft of the radius.
   Angle *2* = The angle of intersection of EF and GH measured anteriorly.

3. *Source of Material*

   The data are based on a study of 50 normal adult subjects, equally divided between
   males and females ranging in age from 18 to 75 years.

MEASUREMENT OF WRIST FLEXION AND EXTENSION*

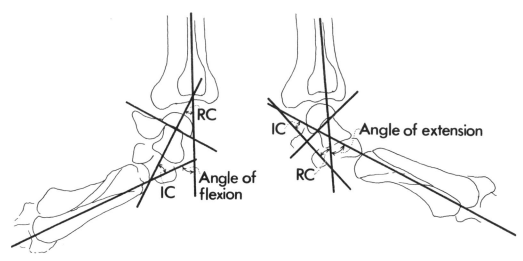

FIG. 123.—(Redrawn from Brumfield *et al.*, Fig. 1.)

1. Technique

    a) Central ray: Perpendicular to plane of film projected over the navicular bone.

    b) Position: True lateral in full flexion, neutral and full extension.

    c) Target-film distance: Immaterial.

2. Measurements

    See Figure 123.

    a) The longitudinal axes of radius and second metacarpal are drawn. The angles are measured as shown in Figure 123. Total wrist motion is flexion plus extension.

    b) The main axes of the lunate are determined by a line on the intercarpal face and a second line drawn at 90° to the first line.

    c) The radiocarpal angle *(RC)* and intercarpal angle *(IC)* are drawn as shown in Figure 123.

	Extension	Flexion	Average Values Total Motion	Radiocarpal	Intercarpal
Males	72°	79°	151°	60°	77°
Females	72°	84°	156°	65°	82°

3. Source of Material

Ten healthy adults between 25 and 35 years of age.

*Brumfield, R. H.; Nickel, V. L.; and Nickel, E.: South. Med. J. 59:909, 1966.

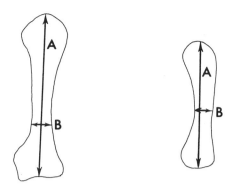

SECOND METACARPAL   FIFTH METACARPAL

FIG. 124.

1. *Technique*

   a) Central ray: Perpendicular to plane of film centered over palm.
   b) Position: Posteroanterior.
   c) Target-film distance: 30 inches.

2. *Measurements*

   See Figure 124.
   a) Axial length: Place a ruler along center line of the shaft of the bone so that the shaft is divided into two equal parts. Measurement *A*, Figure 124.
   b) Minimal width of shaft: Measurement *B*, Figure 124.
   c) Metacarpal Index is calculated by measuring the 2nd, 3rd, 4th and 5th metacarpals. The sum of lengths *(A)* is divided by the sum of widths *(B)*.

Metacarpal Index During First 2 Years

Age (mth.)	Sex	Mean	S.D.
6	M	5.23	0.46
	F	5.60	0.37
12	M	5.30	0.41
	F	5.75	0.41
18	M	5.28	0.40
	F	5.82	0.45
24	M	5.40	0.43
	F	5.84	0.43

(From Joseph and Meadow, Table 1.)

Patients with Marfan's syndrome had a metacarpal index of 7 or greater. In mongols the metacarpal index is within normal limits.

3. *Source of Material*

   Radiographs of both hands of 25 girls and 25 boys were taken at ages 6 months, 12 months, 18 months and 24 months. The children were examined, were known to be healthy and had been studied by Dr. Alice Stewart, Oxford University.

---

*Joseph, M. C., and Meadow, S. R.: Arch. Dis. Childhood 44:515, 1969.

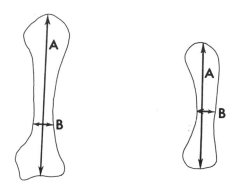

SECOND METACARPAL   FIFTH METACARPAL

FIG. 125.

1. *Technique*

   a) Central ray: Perpendicular to plane of film centered over palm.
   b) Position: Posteroanterior.
   c) Target-film distance: 30 inches.

2. *Measurements*

   See Figure 125.
   a) Axial length: Place a ruler along the center line of the shaft of the bone so that the shaft is divided into two equal parts. Measurement *A*, Figure 125.
   b) Minimal width of shaft: Measurement *B*, Figure 125.
   c) Relative slenderness of each bone = *A/B*.
   d) Metacarpal index is calculated by measuring the 2nd, 3rd, 4th and 5th metacarpals. The sum of lengths *(A)* is divided by the sum of widths *(B)*.

*Parish, J. G.: Brit. J. Radiol. 39:52, 1966.

MALE RIGHT HAND:LENGTH, WIDTH AND RELATIVE SLENDERNESS OF METACARPALS, AND METACARPAL INDEX

		Mean (mm.)	Range (mm.)	Standard Deviation	Coefficient of Variability*
					%
Right metacarpal 1.	Length	46.20	41-55	±2.9	6.3
	Width	10.98	8.5-13.0	±1.03	9.4
	Rel. slend.	4.25	3.6-5.2	±0.42	9.9
Right metacarpal 2.	Length	68.60	57-79	±3.8	5.5
	Width	9.47	8.0-11.5	±0.76	8.0
	Rel. slend.	7.29	6.0-8.6	±0.61	8.4
Right metacarpal 3.	Length	66.40	59-75	±3.2	4.8
	Width	9.31	8.0-10.5	±0.68	7.3
	Rel. slend.	7.16	6.3-8.1	±0.50	7.0
Right metacarpal 4.	Length	59.40	51-65	+3.0	5.1
	Width	7.61	6.5-9.0	±0.58	7.6
	Rel. slend.	7.85	6.4-9.2	±0.63	8.0
Right metacarpal 5.	Length	55.30	49-61	±2.7	4.9
	Width	9.01	7.5-10.5	±0.76	8.4
	Rel. slend.	6.18	5.0-7.7	±0.57	9.2
Right metacarpal index		6.86	5.9 8.1	±0.45	6.6

*Coefficient of variability = (S.D./Mean) × 100.

FIG. 126.—(From Parish, Table II.)

MALE LEFT HAND: LENGTH, WIDTH AND RELATIVE SLENDERNESS OF METACARPALS, AND METACARPAL INDEX

		Mean (mm.)	Range (mm.)	Standard Deviation	Coefficient of Variability
					%
Left metacarpal 1.	Length	46.20	40-54	±3.1	6.7
	Width	10.93	9.5-13.0	±0.88	8.1
	Rel. slend.	4.24	3.5-5.1	±0.36	8.5
Left metacarpal 2.	Length	68.60	63-78	±3.4	5.0
	Width	9.34	8.0-11.0	±0.77	8.2
	Rel. slend.	7.41	6.4-9.1	±0.59	8.0
Left metacarpal 3.	Length	66.50	59-75	±3.2	4.8
	Width	9.22	7.5-10.5	±0.71	7.7
	Rel. slend.	7.25	6.3-9.1	±0.55	7.6
Left metacarpal 4.	Length	59.40	55-66	±3.1	5.2
	Width	7.47	6.5-9.0	±0.56	7.5
	Rel. slend.	7.99	6.9-9.8	±0.60	7.5
Left metacarpal 5.	Length	55.40	49-61	±2.7	4.9
	Width	8.68	7.5-10.0	±0.73	8.4
	Rel. slend.	6.42	5.4-7.7	±0.59	9.2
Left metacarpal index		7.02	6.0-85	±0.49	7.0

FIG. 127.—(From Parish, Table III.)

FEMALE RIGHT HAND: LENGTH, WIDTH AND RELATIVE SLENDERNESS OF METACARPALS, AND METACARPAL INDEX

		Mean (mm.)	Range (mm.)	Standard Deviation	Coefficient of Variability
					%
Right metacarpal 1.	Length	42.70	37-49	±2.3	5.4
	Width	9.04	7.5-11.0	±0.74	8.2
	Rel. slend.	4.74	3.8-6.1	±0.42	8.9
Right metacarpal 2.	Length	64.40	58-74	±3.2	5.0
	Width	8.02	6.5-9.5	±0.62	7.7
	Rel. slend.	8.06	6.7-9.2	±0.63	7.8
Right metacarpal 3.	Length	62.00	57-69	±3.1	5.0
	Width	8.03	6.5-9.5	±0.62	7.7
	Rel. slend.	7.76	6.4-9.1	±0.62	8.0
Right metacarpal 4.	Length	55.60	50-61	±2.8	5.0
	Width	6.38	5.0-7.5	±0.55	8.6
	Rel. slend.	8.78	7.2-10.7	±0.83	9.5
Right metacarpal 5.	Length	51.50	46-57	±2.5	4.9
	Width	7.35	6.0-9.0	±0.61	8.3
	Rel. slend.	7.05	5.4-8.8	±0.63	8.9
Right metacarpal index		7.60	6.3-8.9	±0.52	6.8

FIG. 128.—(From Parish, Table VIII.)

FEMALE LEFT HAND: LENGTH, WIDTH AND RELATIVE SLENDERNESS OF METACARPALS, AND METACARPAL INDEX

		Mean (mm.)	Range (mm.)	Standard Deviation	Coefficient of Variability
					%
Left metacarpal 1.	Length	42.40	37-49	±2.3	5.4
	Width	9.04	7.5-11.0	±0.71	7.9
	Rel. slend.	4.71	4.0-5.9	±0.42	8.9
Left metacarpal 2.	Length	64.00	58-73	±3.1	4.8
	Width	7.90	6.5-9.0	±0.57	7.2
	Rel. slend.	8.13	6.9-9.7	±0.60	7.4
Left metacarpal 3.	Length	61.70	56-70	±3.1	5.0
	Width	7.87	7.0-9.0	±0.53	6.7
	Rel. slend.	7.87	6.7-9.4	±0.53	6.7
Left metacarpal 4.	Length	55.20	50-61	±2.8	5.1
	Width	6.13	5.0-7.0	±0.51	8.3
	Rel. slend.	9.05	7.6-10.9	±0.80	8.8
Left metacarpal 5.	Length	51.10	46-57	±2.5	4.9
	Width	7.10	6.0-9.0	±0.65	9.2
	Rel. slend.	7.25	5.2-8.7	±0.67	9.2
Left metacarpal index		7.78	6.8-9.0	±0.49	6.3

FIG. 129.—(From Parish, Table IX.)

The metacarpal index is above the normal range in arachnodactyly and below normal in Morquio's disease, Weill-Marchesani syndrome and familial streblodactyly. Parish suggests for arachnodactyly a dividing line between normal and abnormal at the 3 S.D. level of 8.4 in males and 9.2 in females.

3. *Source of Material*

Eighty-two female and 51 male patients between the ages of 21 and 45 years who were seen in the physical medicine department of Dryburn Hospital, Durham, England. Patients exhibiting bone or joint disease or congenital abnormalities of the skeletal system were excluded from the study.

RELATIVE PROPORTIONS OF THE BONES OF THE THUMB*

1. Technique

   a) Central ray: Perpendicular to plane of film projected over palm.
   b) Position: Posteroanterior.
   c) Target-film distance: Immaterial.

2. Measurements

See Figure 125.

Measurements are made along the axis of each bone and the maximum length is used.

The ratio approach is more useful than comparisons with normal standards for length because it is not dependent on the size of the individual and a relative disproportion in length of bones is more easily detected.

3. Source of Material

Measurements are from the studies of Garn at Fels Research Institute, Yellow Springs, Ohio.

---

*Poznanski, A. K.; Garn, S. M.; and Holt, J. F.: Radiology. 100:115, 1971.

RELATIVE PROPORTIONS OF THE BONES OF THE THUMB

		MALES				FEMALES			
		Diaphysis and Epiphysis			Diaph- ysis	Diaphysis and Epiphysis			Diaph- ysis
		Adult	9 Yr.	4 Yr.	1 Yr.	Adult	9 Yr.	4 Yr.	1 Yr.
Met 2/Met 1	Mean	1.49	1.53	1.57	1.64	1.52	1.52	1.55	1.60
	S.D.	0.05	0.05	0.06	0.06	0.07	0.06	0.07	0.09
Met 2/P 1	Mean	2.10	2.28	2.22	2.13	2.13	2.25	2.22	2.15
	S.D.	0.10	0.12	0.11	0.11	0.12	0.13	0.11	0.13
Met 2/D 1	Mean	2.93	2.93	2.88	2.85	3.02	2.96	2.90	2.89
	S.D.	0.16	0.15	0.16	0.18	0.20	0.16	0.14	0.19
Met 1/Met 2	Mean	0.67	0.66	0.64	0.61	0.66	0.66	0.65	0.63
	S.D.	0.02	0.02	0.02	0.02	0.04	0.03	0.03	0.04
Met 1/P 1	Mean	1.41	1.49	1.41	1.31	1.41	1.49	1.44	1.34
	S.D.	0.06	0.06	0.06	0.06	0.05	0.07	0.06	0.07
Met 1/D 1	Mean	1.97	1.92	1.82	1.74	1.99	1.95	1.88	1.81
	S.D.	0.12	0.10	0.10	0.10	0.12	0.11	0.11	0.14
P 1/Met 2	Mean	0.48	0.44	0.45	0.47	0.47	0.45	0.45	0.47
	S.D.	0.02	0.02	0.02	0.02	0.03	0.02	0.02	0.03
P 1/Met 1	Mean	0.71	0.67	0.71	0.77	0.71	0.67	0.70	0.75
	S.D.	0.03	0.03	0.03	0.04	0.03	0.03	0.03	0.04
P 1/D 1	Mean	1.40	1.29	1.30	1.34	1.42	1.32	1.31	1.35
	S.D.	0.08	0.07	0.07	0.08	0.09	0.08	0.07	0.09
D 1/Met 2	Mean	0.34	0.34	0.35	0.35	0.33	0.34	0.35	0.35
	S.D.	0.02	0.02	0.02	0.02	0.02	0.02	0.02	0.02
D 1/Met 1	Mean	0.51	0.52	0.55	0.58	0.50	0.51	0.53	0.56
	S.D.	0.03	0.03	0.03	0.03	0.03	0.03	0.03	0.04
D 1/P 1	Mean	0.72	0.78	0.77	0.75	0.71	0.76	0.77	0.75
	S.D.	0.04	0.04	0.04	0.04	0.04	0.05	0.04	0.05

Met 1 = Metacarpal of the thumb P 1 = Proximal phalanx of the thumb
Met 2 = Second metacarpal D 1 = Distal phalanx of the thumb

FIG. 130.—(From Poznanski, Table 1.)

MEASUREMENT OF COMBINED CORTICAL THICKNESS (C.C.T.) OF METACARPAL* AND HUMERUS† IN CHILDREN AND ADULTS

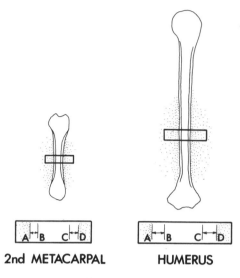

2nd METACARPAL   **HUMERUS**

C.C. T. = AB + CD

FIG. 131.

1. *Technique*

    a) Central ray: Metacarpal—Perpendicular to plane of film projected over palm.
                        Humerus—Perpendicular to plane of film centered over lower third
                           of humerus.
    b) Position: Metacarpal—Posteroanterior.
                     Humerus—Anteroposterior.
    c) Target-film distance: Metacarpal—36 inches.
                             Humerus—42 inches.

2. *Measurements*

    a) Second metacarpal (right or left). See Figure 131.
        Measurements made at midshaft.
        C.C.T. = Shaft width *(T)*—Medullary width *(M)*.
    b) Female humerus (left). See Figure 131.
        Measurements are made at the most distal point on the shaft of the bone where
        the endosteal borders of the lateral and medial cortices are parallel to each
        other and to the outer margins of the cortices. This is usually about 10–12 cm.
        from the most distal end of the bone.
            The combined cortical thickness (C.C.T.) is the sum of the medial and
        lateral cortices.
    c) Age-dependent variations of C.C.T. of 2nd right metacarpal bone in males.‡

---

*Garn, S. E.: *The Earlier Gain and the Later Loss of Cortical Bone in Nutritional Perspective* (Springfield, Ill.: Charles C. Thomas, Publisher, 1970), Table 2.

†Bloom, R. A., and Laws, J. W.: Brit. J. Radiol. 43:522, 1970.

‡Virtama, P., and Helelä, T.: Acta radiol., supp. 293, 1969.

MEASUREMENT OF COMBINED CORTICAL THICKNESS (C.C.T.) OF METACARPAL AND HUMERUS IN CHILDREN AND ADULTS

a) Second metacarpal (right or left). See Figure 131.

Age	Total Width (T) (mm.)		Medullary Width (M) (mm.)		Cortical Width (C.C.T.) (mm.)	
	Mean	S.D.	Mean	S.D.	Mean	S.D.
			Males			
1	4.50	0.34	3.04	0.45	1.46	0.30
2	5.11	0.44	3.24	0.62	1.85	0.39
4	5.53	0.49	3.04	0.62	2.48	0.37
6	6.05	0.53	3.06	0.66	2.98	0.44
8	6.57	0.54	3.13	0.66	3.43	0.45
10	7.16	0.59	3.28	0.66	3.88	0.49
12	7.73	0.65	3.43	0.72	4.29	0.60
14	8.52	0.77	3.63	0.72	4.89	0.68
16	9.11	0.72	3.81	0.75	5.29	0.51
18	9.31	0.68	3.56	0.90	5.75	0.66
30	9.36	0.68	3.41	0.81	5.94	0.43
40	9.35	0.50	3.72	0.83	5.63	0.60
50	9.65	0.88	3.84	0.93	5.81	0.63
60	9.69	0.62	4.44	0.04	5.24	0.62
70	9.38	0.58	4.61	1.05	4.76	0.73
80	9.07	0.51	4.23	0.62	4.89	0.56
			Females			
1	4.35	0.36	2.87	0.38	1.47	0.31
2	4.91	0.47	3.12	0.53	1.79	0.36
4	5.37	0.49	3.04	0.49	2.32	0.35
6	5.76	0.53	3.01	0.51	2.76	0.43
8	6.26	0.58	3.05	0.58	3.20	0.41
10	6.80	0.63	3.26	0.64	3.53	0.48
12	7.40	0.68	3.25	0.74	4.14	0.57
14	7.77	0.62	2.94	0.68	4.83	0.57
16	7.79	0.61	2.71	0.71	5.08	0.60
18	7.90	0.64	2.71	0.72	5.18	0.68
30	7.94	0.55	2.61	0.80	5.33	0.69
40	8.08	0.65	2.59	0.89	5.45	0.81
50	7.79	0.66	2.27	0.71	5.52	0.75
60	8.12	0.43	3.26	0.88	4.85	0.68
70	8.34	0.70	4.38	0.88	3.99	0.63
80	8.29	0.61	5.00	0.64	3.30	0.51

FIG. 132.—(From Garn,* Table 3.)

*Garn, S. E.; Poznanski, A. K.; and Nagy, J. M.: Radiology 100:509, 1971.

b) Female humerus (left). See Figure 131.

Age Group	Mean C.C.T.	S.D.
Teens	8.65	0.90
20-29	8.60	0.80
30-39	9.00	0.75
40-49	8.90	0.80
50-54	8.35	1.00
55-59	7.95	1.26
60-64	7.25	1.30
65-69	6.60	1.25
70-74	6.50	1.10
75-79	5.75	1.20
80+	5.50	0.75

(From Bloom and Laws, Table 1.)

c) Dependent variations of C.C.T. of second right metacarpal bone in males.

FIG. 133.—(From Virtama and Helelä, Fig. 3.)

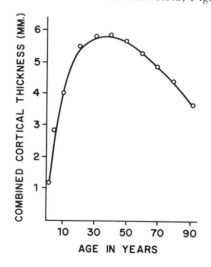

3. Source of Material

a) Metacarpal measurements are from 734 patients in Garn's extensive studies on growth.

b) Humerus measurements are from 254 unselected female patients, King's College Hospital, London.

   Note:
   Virtama and Helelä have published the results of their extensive studies on combined cortical thickness in which 34 bone sites were measured in females and males between ages 1 year and 90 years living in southwestern Finland. Figure 133 shows an example of variation in C.C.T. with age. Virtama and Helelä compared their results with those from Fels Research Institute for Human Development, Yellow Springs, Ohio, and concluded that the amount of cortical bone in the Finnish population is lower than that in the Ohio population.

E. The Pelvis and Hip

AXIAL RELATIONSHIPS OF THE HIP JOINT*

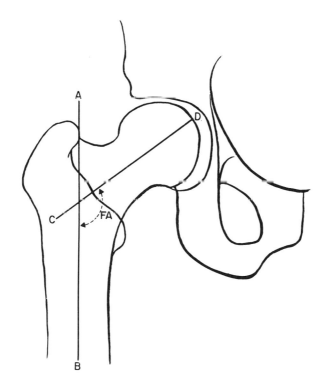

FIG. 134.

Angle *FA:*

    Males   128°
    Females 127°

*Keats, T. E., *et al.:* Radiology 87:904, 1966.

AXIAL RELATIONSHIPS OF THE HIP JOINT

1. Technique

a) Central ray: Passes through a point 1 inch below the center of the inguinal ligament perpendicular to the plane of the film.

b) Position: Anteroposterior. The patient is placed flat on his back with the toe of the foot pointing somewhat to the median plane.

c) Target-film distance: Immaterial.

2. Measurements

See Figure 134.

AB = Line along midaxis of femoral shaft.
CD = Line along midaxis of femoral head and neck.
Angle FA = Angle of the femoral neck at intersection of AB and CD.

3. Source of Material

The data are based on a study of 50 normal adult subjects, equally divided between male and female ranging in age from 19 to 76 years.

WIDTH OF THE HIP JOINT SPACE*

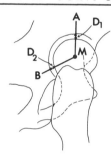

FIG. 135.—(Redrawn from Zwicker *et al.*, Diagram 1.)

1. Technique

a) Central ray: To greater trochanter of femur perpendicular to the plane of the film.

b) Position: Anteroposterior. Oblique of pelvis with hip elevated and with internal rotation of the femur to project the greater trochanter over the neck of the femur as shown in Figure 135.

c) Target-film distance: 150 cm.

2. Measurements

See Figure 135.

MA = Line from midpoint of head of femur to superior margin of acetabulum.
MB = Line from midpoint of head of femur to medial and inferior margin of acetabulum.

Average Joint Space Width

D_1	S.D.	D_2	S.D.
3.0 mm.	0.28 mm.	4.0 mm.	0.53 mm.

3. Source of Material

Twenty-six normal adult patients.

---

*Zwicker, H.; Münzenberg, K. J.; and Düx, A.: Fortschr. Geb. Röntgenstrahlen 111:693, 1969.

MEASUREMENT OF PROTUSIO ACETABULI*

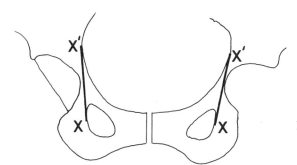

FIG. 136.—(Redrawn from Hubbard, Fig. 1.)

1. *Technique*

   a) Central ray: Perpendicular to plane of film centered over midpelvis.

   b) Position: Anteroposterior.

   c) Target-film distance: Immaterial.

2. *Measurements*

   See Figure 136.

   The outline of the dome of the acetabulum meets Köhler's line $X'X$. This line is drawn from the pelvic border of the ilium to the medial border of the body of the ischium.

   If the outline of the acetabular dome passes medial to line $X'X$, a protrusion exists.

   This method is applicable to serial roentgenograms of an individual patient and is not suitable for comparing patients.

3. *Source of Material*

   The data are from 242 patients with a diagnosis of degenerative arthritis of the hip.

---

*Hubbard, M. J. S.: Am. J. Roentgenol. 106:506, 1969.

THE ACETABULAR ANGLE OF THE GROWING HIP*

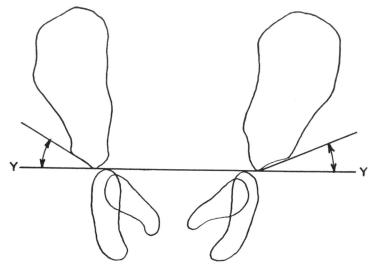

FIG. 137.

COMPARISON OF ACETABULAR ANGLES AT DIFFERENT
AGES IN ALL CATEGORIES[†]

	MEAN VALUES (Degrees)			2-S.D. RANGE (Degrees)		
	Newborn	6 Mo.	12 Mo.	Newborn	6 Mo.	12 Mo.
White:						
Male:						
Right	25.8	19.4	19.1	34-17	26-12	26-12
Left	27.0	20.9	20.6	37-17	28-13	28-13
Female:						
Right	28.3	22.1	20.5	38-18	30-14	28-13
Left	29.4	23.4	21.9	39-20	32-15	29-14
Negro:						
Male:						
Right	24.8	21.4	20.5	34-15	31-12	29-12
Left	26.0	23.0	21.9	36-16	32-14	30-14
Female:						
Right	27.7	23.9	22.5	38-18	32-16	30-15
Left	29.4	25.4	24.4	39-19	33-18	32-16

[†]Adapted from Caffey *et al.*, Table 4, p. 639.

*Caffey, J.; Ames, R.; Silverman, W. A.; Ryder, C. T.; and Hough, G.: Pediatrics 17:632, 1956.

THE ACETABULAR ANGLE OF THE GROWING HIP

1. *Technique*

   a) Central ray: Perpendicular to plane of film centered to a point about 1 inch superior to the pubic symphysis.

   b) Position: Anteroposterior.

   c) Target-film distance: Immaterial.

2. *Measurements*

   See Figure 137.

   The acetabular angle is formed between a transverse line drawn through the right and left *Y* cartilages in the iliums (the *Y-Y* line) and an oblique line connecting the medial and lateral ends of the bony edge behind and above the acetabular face.

   There are small differences in the left and right acetabular angles in all categories of patients (see table below Figure 137). There is also a distinct difference in size of the angles on both sides in females and males.

   Congenital dislocation of the hip is all but unknown in Negroes.

3. *Source of Material*

   The radiologic findings were derived from 627 newborn infants, of whom 551 were later re-examined at 6 months and 527 at 12 months. This study did not include premature, mongols, children whose hips dislocated under observations, or children whose racial origins could not be determined accurately.

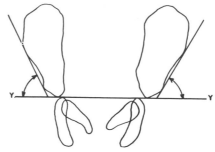

FIG. 138.

Category	Mean	SD	2 SD Range	Actual Range
Acetabular Angles in Degrees				
Younger Mongoloids	16	4.5	25–7	29–9
Younger Normals	28	4.7	37–18	44–12
Older Mongoloids	11	4.2	19–3	19–6
Older Normals	22	4.2	8–14	34–8
Iliac Angles in Degrees				
Younger Mongoloids	44	6.5	56–30	58–35
Younger Normals	55	5.5	66–44	67–43
Older Mongoloids	41	7.0	55–29	50–26
Older Normals	58	7.0	72–43	74–44
Iliac Indices				
Younger Mongoloids	60	9.9	80–49	87–48
Younger Normals	81	8.0	97–65	97–68
Older Mongoloids	50	9.6	67–29	67–33
Older Normals	79	9.0	96–60	101–62

"Younger" means younger than 3 months; "older" means 3-12 months of age. (From Caffey and Ross, Table 2.)

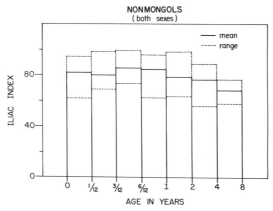

Variation of the normal iliac index with age. (Redrawn from Astley.[†])

*Caffey, J., and Ross, S.: Am. J. Roentgenol. 80:458, 1958.
[†]Astley, R.: Brit. J. Radiol. 36:2, 1963.

THE ILIAC ANGLE AND THE ILIAC INDEX OF THE GROWING HIP

1. Technique

 a) Central ray: Perpendicular to plane of film centered to a point about 1 inch superior to the pubic symphysis.

 b) Position: Anteroposterior.

 c) Target-film distance: Immaterial.

2. Measurements

See Figure 138.

The iliac angle is formed between a line drawn through the lower edges of the *Y* cartilages (the *Y-Y* line) and the oblique lines drawn through two points, the most lateral point of the iliac body below and the most lateral point on the iliac wing above.

The iliac index is a combination of the iliac angle and the acetabular angle and may prove more useful than either single measurement. The iliac index is the sum of both acetabular angles and both iliac angles divided by 2. These measurements are useful in the diagnosis of mongolism, where low values are obtained.

Astley states that, if the iliac index is under 60, mongolism is very possible. If it is over 78, the child is probably normal. If it lies in between, only a qualified report can be given. If the index is between 68 and 60, mongolism is probable; but a note must be added that 10% of normals occur in this range. If the index is between 68 and 78, the child is probably not a mongol, but a notation must be added that 6% of mongols do occur in this range.

3. Source of Material

Caffey and Ross's data are based on a study of 48 mongoloid infants who varied in age from 2 days to 12 months and on a previous study of 1,500 unselected newborn infants in whom the pelvis and hips were examined roentgenographically.

Astley's study is based on 106 nonmongol children from birth to 8 years and on 34 children in whom there was a clinical question of mongolism.

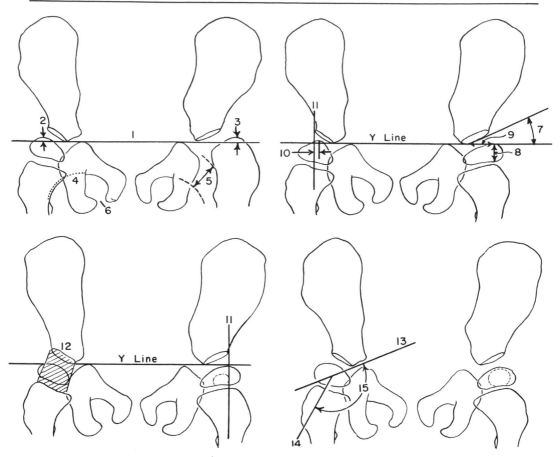

FIG. 139.—(Redrawn from Meschan, I.: *Roentgen Signs in Clinical Diagnosis* [Philadelphia: W. B. Saunders Company, 1956].)

*Kohler, A., and Zimmer, E. A.: *Borderlands of the Normal and Early Pathologic in Skeletal Roentgenology* (English trans. by J. T. Case) (New York: Grune & Stratton, Inc., 1956), pp. 491-494.

CRITERIA FOR DETECTION OF ABNORMALITY OF THE GROWING HIP

1. Technique

    a) Central ray: Passes through a point 1 inch below the center of the inguinal ligament, perpendicular to the plane of the film.

    b) Position: Anteroposterior. The patient is placed flat on his back with the toe of the foot pointing somewhat to the median plane.

    c) Target-film distance: Immaterial.

2. Measurements

    See Figure 139.

        1 = Y symphysial line, drawn horizontally through the cotyloid notches of the acetabula.

        2 and *3* = Distances from the apex of the femoral head to the Y symphysial line *(1)*. Normally, these distances are equal.

        4 = Shenton's line. Follows the upper arched contour of the obturator foramen, thus marking the lower margin of the pubic bone, and is continued as a regularly curved line into the lower border of the femoral neck.

        5 = Break in continuity of Shenton's line, indicating dislocation or fracture.

        6 = Fusion of the ischiopubic synchondrosis—may be delayed with dislocation.

        7 = The angle of the acetabulum, the angle formed between a line from the cotyloid notch on the Y symphysial line to the superior acetabular lip on that side. If this angle is more than 34° in the newborn or more than 25° in a child a year old, it may be said that a "steep acetabular roof" is present. (See also the section on the acetabular angle, page 126.)

        8 = The diaphysial interval, the distance between the diaphysis of the femur (which is conical in the period before ossification of the femoral head) and the Y symphysial line. This distance should not be less than 6 cm.

        9 = If in the newborn the distance of the pivotal point (point of intersection of line *8* and the Y symphysial line) from the tip of the acetabular angle is more than 16 mm., the presence of a luxation, must be suspected.

        10 = This is the horizontal distance between the vertical line of Ombrédanne (see *11*) and line *8*. This distance is normally less than one half of the epiphysial width (not illustrated).

        11 = The vertical line of Ombrédanne, which intersects the upper jutting edge of the acetabular roof and is perpendicular to the Y symphysial line. The center of ossification of the normal femoral head lies below the horizontal line and medial to the vertical line; in cases of luxation, this center will be above and lateral, respectively.

        12 = The parallelogram of Köpitz. A very near approach to a right angle is normal; the head of the femur will be found very close to the center. In cases of luxation of the hip, a rhomboid will be observed and the head of the femur will have an eccentric position.

        13 = The guide line of the Y symphysis down from the center of the acetabulum to the center of the head.

        14 = The axis of the neck of the femur.

        15 = The angle between *13* and *14*, normally 120°-125°.

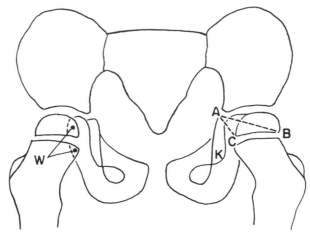

FIG. 140.–(Redrawn from Meschan, I.: *Roentgen Signs in Clinical Diagnosis* [Philadelphia: W. B. Saunders Company, 1956].)

See Figure 140.

WW = Waldenström's overlap, a crescentic shadow formed by the overlapping of the medial quadrant of the femoral head on the posterior lip of the acetabulum. In normal hips the overlap shadows are of equal size. If an inflammatory process is present or an acetabular aclivity exists, the femoral head on that side will be pushed laterally, diminishing the width of the overlap shadow.

K = Köhler's teardrop, the end-on view of the lower anterior acetabular floor. The teardrops should be symmetrical bilaterally. See also page 135.

ABC = Triangle formed by lines drawn from the cotyloid notch to both margins of the femoral epiphysial line. The sides of the triangle should coincide with the triangle of the opposite hip. Inequality of the two triangles is an early indication of anatomic imbalance and hip-joint pathology.

*Martin, H. E.: Radiology 56:842, 1951.

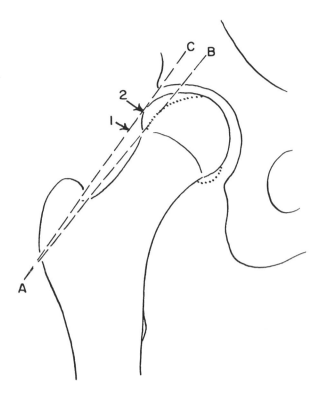

FIG. 141.—(Redrawn from Martin, Fig. 6.)

See Figure 141.

AB = Line intersecting a superior lateral segment of the femoral head.

AC = Line tangential to the arc of the femoral head. When slipping occurs *(dotted line)*, the head descends and the neck rides upward. Line *AC* therefore disappears, to overlie line *AB*, which is now a tangential line on the femoral head rather than an intersecting line.

1 and *2* = Arrows indicating the usual concavoconvexity at the superior epiphysial junction.

3. *Source of Material*

These measurements were derived from the work of many investigators. The reader will find an extensive bibliography to these sources in Köhler's book[†] and in the article by Martin.

*Martin, H. E.: Radiology 56:842, 1951; also Watson-Jones, R.: *Fractures and Joint Injuries* (4th ed.; Baltimore: Williams & Wilkins Company, 1955), Vol. 2, p. 658 (quoted by Martin).

[†]Köhler, A., and Zimmer, E. A.: *Borderlands of the Normal and Early Pathologic in Skeletal Roentgenology* (English trans. by J. T. Case) (New York: Grune & Stratton, Inc., 1956), pp. 491-494.

DETECTION OF CONGENITAL DISLOCATION OF THE HIP BEFORE APPEARANCE OF CAPITAL FEMORAL EPIPHYSIS*

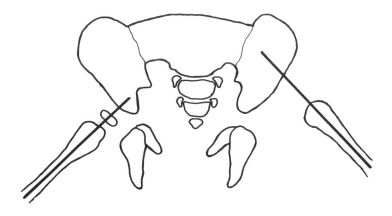

FIG. 142.

1. *Technique*

   a) Central ray: Projected over midpelvis perpendicular to plane of film.

   b) Position: Anteroposterior supine. The femora are abducted forcibly to at least 45° with appreciable inward rotation of the femora.

   c) Target-film distance: Immaterial.

2. *Measurements*

   See Figure 142.

   The manipulation displaces the head medially, with the result that it is forced either into or out of the socket, depending on the presence or absence of dislocation, so that the head never assumes an intermediate position. If the hip is normal, the line of the femoral shaft will be directed toward the upper edge of the bony acetabular wall; but in the presence of congenital dislocation of the hip, it will point to the anterior superior iliac spine. Abduction should be 45° or more; otherwise, the roentgenograms may be misleading. A fair degree of inward rotation is also necessary because of the marked antetorsion of the femoral necks in newborns.

3. *Source of Material*

   This method is based on a study of 15,373 newborns, in which 14 cases of congenital dislocation of the hip were found (0.1%).

---

*Andren, L., and Von Rosen, S.: Acta radiol. 49:89, 1958.

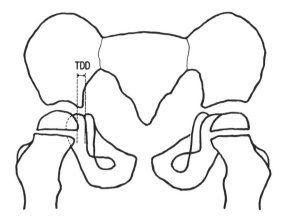

FIG. 143.

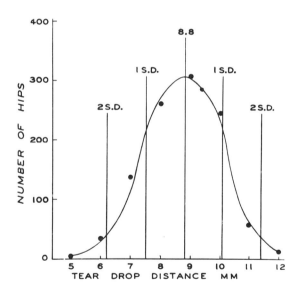

(From Eyring *et al.*, Fig. 11.*)

*Eyring, E. J., *et al.*: Am. J. Roentgenol. 93:382, 1965.

EARLY DETECTION OF PERTHES' DISEASE – THE TEARDROP DISTANCE

1. *Technique*

   a) Central ray: Perpendicular to plane of film centered over midpelvis.

   b) Position: Anteroposterior. Positioning does not alter the measurement, provided the femur is not rotated internally or externally more than 30°, flexed more than 30°, or abducted more than 15°.

   c) Target-film distance: 40 inches.

2. *Measurements*

   See Figure 143.

   Measurement is made from the lateral margin of the pelvic teardrop to the medial border of the proximal femoral metaphysis. Measurements are independent of the age of the subject. The teardrop distance *(TDD)*, when greater than 11 mm., or more than 2 mm. greater than that of the opposite hip, is a sensitive indicator of hip joint disease.

3. *Source of Material*

   The data are based on a study of 1,070 normal hips of persons from 1 to 11 years and on 49 hips affected by Perthes' disease.

F. The Lower Extremity

MEASUREMENT OF THE DEGREE OF ANTEVERSION OF THE FEMORAL NECK

Direct Method of Budin and Chandler*

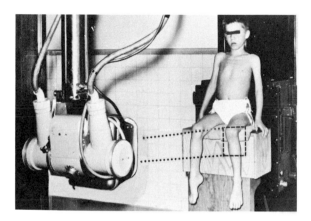

FIG. 144.—Position of patient in relation to the x-ray tube, showing approximate size of field. (From Budin and Chandler, Fig. 1.)

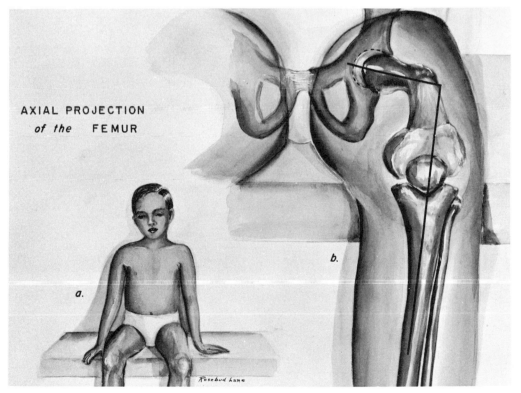

FIG. 145.—Axial view of femur, showing axis of the neck and tibial reference line. (From Budin and Chandler, Fig. 2.)

*Budin, E., and Chandler, E.: Radiology 69:209, 1957.

MEASUREMENT OF THE DEGREE OF ANTEVERSION
OF THE FEMORAL NECK

Direct Method of Budin and Chandler

1. Technique

  a) Central ray: Projected along the axis of the femur, with the patient being rotated as is necessary. The beam is centered on the femoral neck (Fig. 144).

  b) Position: The patient sits with knees flexed close to 90° on a wooden box which has been placed on the footrest of the vertical x-ray table. In limiting the field size, it is important to include the upper third of the tibia on the film as a reference line (Figs. 145 and 147), and yet narrow the field so that the gonads are completely shielded from the primary beam of radiation. This can be checked with boys by using a light-beam localizer; for girls, a field 2 inches wide is adequate. The use of a lead shield to cover the gonads will provide further protection. Repetition of examination should be avoided.

  c) Target-film distance: 48 inches.
  Technical factors: 100 ma, 6 seconds, 90-100 kvp. Because of the high ma value, this procedure probably should not be attempted on children over 6 years of age unless they are unusually thin.

2. Measurements

This method consists of visualizing the femur in the true axial projection, with the coronal plane (or the bicondylar plane) defined by the axis of the flexed tibia, which is perpendicular to it. Only one plane is perpendicular to a line. It can be readily shown geometrically that the projection of the long axis of the tibia in any degree of flexion is always perpendicular to the bicondylar plane. Thus the actual angle which the femoral neck makes with the coronal plane is directly recorded on the film. This is illustrated in Figure 146, *A*, where the horizontal line is perpendicular to the axis of the tibia and the angle of anteversion is the angle formed with this horizontal line by the axis of the femoral head and neck. A constant check on the adequacy of the positioning of the patient is the visualization of the cross-section of the upper femoral shaft on the film when it is taken properly.

3. Source of Material

The figures for normal degrees of anteversion (see table) are averages adapted from reports of four different investigators and include measurements on 259 children and 54 anatomic specimens.

NORMAL DEGREES OF ANTEVERSION, SHOWING PROGRESSION WITH AGE*

AGE	ANTEVERSION (in Degrees)
Birth to 1 yr.	30 - 50
2 yr.	30
3-5 yr.	25
6-12 yr.	20
12-15 yr.	17
16-20 yr.	11
20 yr.	8

*Billing, L.: Acta radiol., supp. 110, 1954. (Averages adapted from several investigators.)

MEASUREMENT OF THE DEGREE OF ANTEVERSION
OF THE FEMORAL NECK

Direct Method of Budin and Chandler

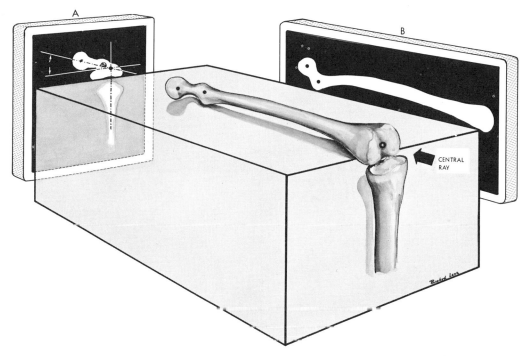

FIG. 146.—Femur and tibia in examining position in relation to central ray. *A*, cassette in position for axial view as projected, with angle of anteversion indicated. *B*, cassette illustrating angle measured on lateral view of femur. (From Budin and Chandler, Fig. 3.)

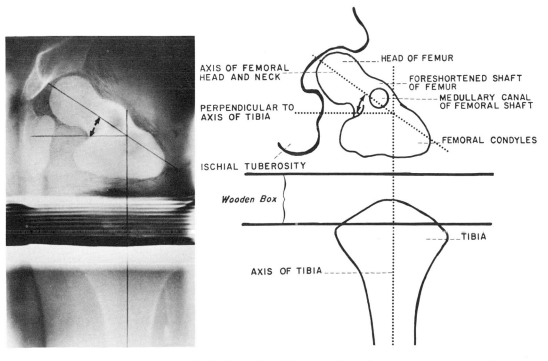

FIG. 147.—Roentgenogram of left femur in axial projection, showing measurement of anteversion, and diagram of anatomic parts seen in film. (From Budin and Chandler, Fig. 4.)

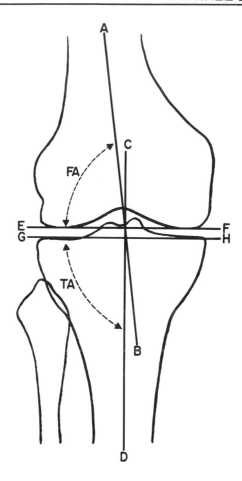

FIG. 148.

	FA	*TA*
Male	75° — 85°	85° — 100°
Female	75° — 85°	87° — 98°
Average	81°	93°

*Keats, T. E., *et al.*: Radiology 87:904, 1966.

AXIAL RELATIONSHIPS OF THE KNEE JOINT

1. *Technique*

   a) Central ray: Passes through a point about 1/2 inch below the tip of the patella, so that it will pass directly through the knee joint space, perpendicular to the plane of the film.

   b.) Position: Anteroposterior.

   c) Target-film distance: Immaterial.

2. *Measurements*

   See Figure 148.

   AB = Line drawn along the midaxis of the femoral shaft.

   CD = Line drawn along the midaxis of the tibial shaft.

   EF = Line tangent to the articular surfaces of the condyles.

   GH = Line tangent to the lateral and medial extremities of the tibial plateau.

   FA = Femoral angle at intersection of AB and EF.

   TA = Tibial angle at intersection of CD and GH.

3. *Source of Material*

   The data were based on a study of 50 normal adult subjects, equally divided between males and females ranging in age from 18 to 66 years.

SAGITTAL PLANE RELATION OF FEMORAL CONDYLES
TO THE LONG AXIS OF THE FEMUR*

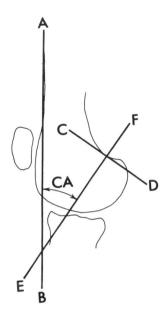

FIG. 149.—(Redrawn from Lindahl and Movin, Fig. 1.)

1. Technique

a) Central ray: Projected through the knee joint space, perpendicular to the plane of the film.
b) Position: True lateral.
c) Target-film distance: Immaterial. (Lindahl used 100 cm.)

2. Measurements

See Figure 149.
AB = Line drawn along the anterior cortical demarcation of shaft of the femur.
CD = Plane for the floor of the intercondylar fossa (the intercondylar plane).
EF = Perpendicular to line CD intersecting line AB.
CA = Angle formed by roof of intercondylar fossa and long axis of femur,

Mean Value	Range
34.0° ± 0.5°	26° to 44°

Right and left sides in same patient showed differences of 0.2° ± 0.2°.

3. Source of Material

Two hundred normal knee joints of 100 patients without knee complaints.

*Lindahl, O., and Movin, A.: Acta radiol. (Diagnosis) 10:108, 1970.

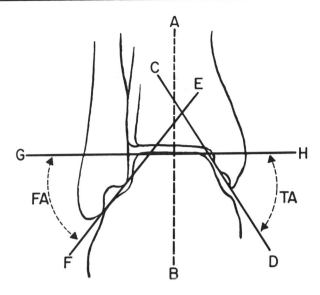

FIG. 150.

	Males	Females	Av.
FA	45° - 63°	43° - 62°	52°
TA	45° - 61°	49° - 65°	53°

*Keats, T. E., *et al.*: Radiology 87:904, 1966.

MEASUREMENT OF THE AXIAL ANGLES OF THE ANKLE

1. *Technique*

    a) Central ray: Perpendicular to plane of film projected through the center of the talotibial joint.

    b) Position: Anteroposterior, with great toe pointing slightly medially.

    c) Target-film distance: Immaterial.

2. *Measurements*

    See Figure 150.

    AB = The axis of the shaft of the tibia. This line is perpendicular to the horizontal plane of the ankle joint and is continuous with the vertical axis of the talus.

    CD = Line tangent to the articular surface of the medial malleolus.

    EF = Line tangent to the articular surface of the lateral malleolus.

    GH = Line tangent to the articular surface of the talus.

    FA = Fibular angle at the intersection of EF and GH.

    TA = Tibial angle at the intersection of CD and GH.

3. *Source of Material*

    The data were based on a study of 50 normal adult subjects, equally divided between males and females ranging in age from 18 to 85 years.

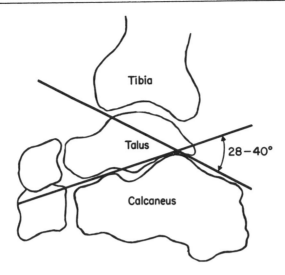

FIG. 151.—Boehler's angle.

1. *Technique*

   a) Central ray: The ankle is placed against the film so that the lateral malleolus is in the central ray.

   b) Position: Lateral. The foot is perpendicular to the film, and the two malleoli should be projected directly over one another.

   c) Target-film distance: Immaterial.

2. *Measurements*

   Boehler's angle (Fig. 151) for the normal calcaneus is formed between a line tangent to the upper contour of the tuberosity of the calcaneus and a line uniting the highest point of the anterior process with the highest point of the posterior articular surface. This angle normally averages 30°-35°. Less than 28° is definitely abnormal and represents poor position.

3. *Source of Material*

   The normal range of this measurement has been derived from radiographs of approximately 1,900 patients who were treated for fracture of the os calcis. In each case, both the normal and injured os calcis were radiographed.

---

*Boehler, L.: J. Bone & Joint Surg. 13:75, 1931.

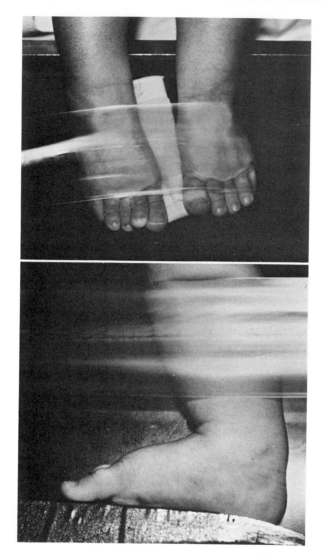

FIG. 152.—Proper positioning of a child's foot for AP and lateral radiographs. A wooden wedge is used on the lateral film to dorsiflex the foot as much as possible and to show the presence or absence of equinas. The position of the bones is not affected by holding the foot in the restrictive plastic strap to procure the anteroposterior view. (Keim, H. A.: Clinical Orthopedics and Related Research 70:133, 1970. Fig. 2.)

*Davis, L. A., and Hatt, W. S.: Radiology 64:818, 1955.

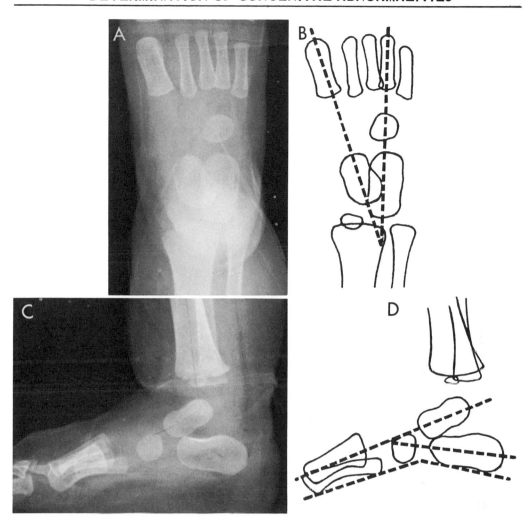

FIG. 153.—Normal foot. *A* and *B*, anteroposterior projection. (1) The angle between the talus and calcaneus varies with age. In infants and young children, the angle is between 30° and 50° (weight bearing). In children older than 5 years, the talocalcaneal angle varies from 15° to 30° (weight bearing). (2) The line through the midtalus points to the head of the 1st metatarsal. (3) The line through the midcalcaneus points to the head of the 4th metatarsal. (4) The midtalar and midcalcaneal lines generally coincide with midshaft lines of the 1st and 4th metatarsals, respectively. (5) Lines of metatarsal shafts are very nearly parallel. *C* and *D*, lateral projection. (1) The midtalar line and the line through the shaft of the 1st metatarsal coincide in children over 5 years of age on weight bearing; but in infants and young children, the talus is positioned more vertically and the midtalar line passes inferiorly to the shaft of the first metatarsal. (2) An obtuse angle is formed by the line through the inferior cortex of the 5th metatarsal, ranging from 150° to 175° (weight bearing). (3) The midtalar line and midcalcaneal line form an acute angle which varies normally from 25° to 50° (weight bearing). (Drawings from Davis and Hatt. Measurements from Templeton, A. W.: Am. J. Roentgenol. 93:374, 1965.)

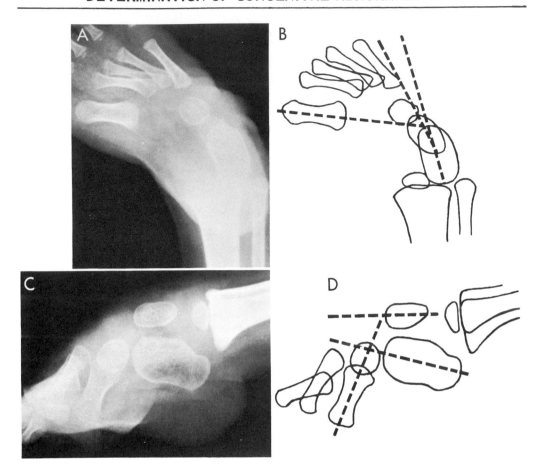

FIG. 154.—Clubfoot. *A* and *B*, anteroposterior projection. (1) The talocalcaneal angle approaches 0° or is even reversed. (2) Midtalar line points lateral to normal position. (3) Midcalcaneal line points lateral to normal position. (4) The midtalar line and the line through the shaft of the 1st metatarsal now form an angle. (5) There is a loss of parallelism of metatarsals, with convergence posteriorly. *C* and *D*, lateral projection. (1) The midtalar line and line through the shaft of the 1st metatarsal form an obtuse angle. (2) Midtalar and midcalcaneal lines approach parallelism. (From Davis and Hatt, Fig. 3.)

AXIAL RELATIONSHIPS OF THE FOOT AND CRITERIA FOR DETERMINATION OF CONGENITAL ABNORMALITIES

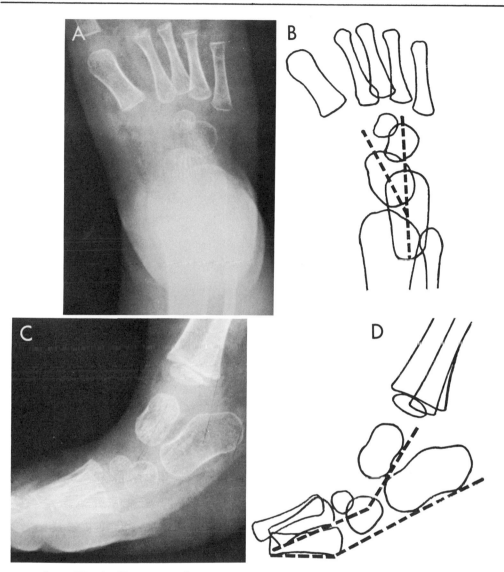

FIG. 155.—"Rocker" deformity (overcorrected clubfoot). *A* and *B*, anteroposterior projection. (1) The angle between the calcaneus and talus is less than average. (2) The forefoot may or may not be normal. *C* and *D*, lateral projection. (1) Reverse angle between inferior cortex of calcaneus and 5th metatarsal. (2) Reverse angle between inferior cortex of talus and 1st metatarsal in severe cases. (From Davis and Hatt, Fig. 4.)

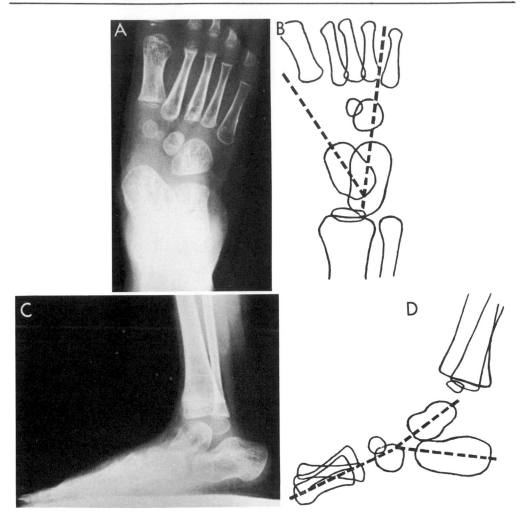

FIG. 156.—Flatfoot. *A* and *B*, anteroposterior. (1) Increased talocalcaneal angle. *C* and *D*, lateral projection. (1) The line of the 1st metatarsal makes an angle instead of coinciding with the midtalar line. (2) Frequently there is an increased talocalcaneal angle. (From Davis and Hatt, Fig. 5.)

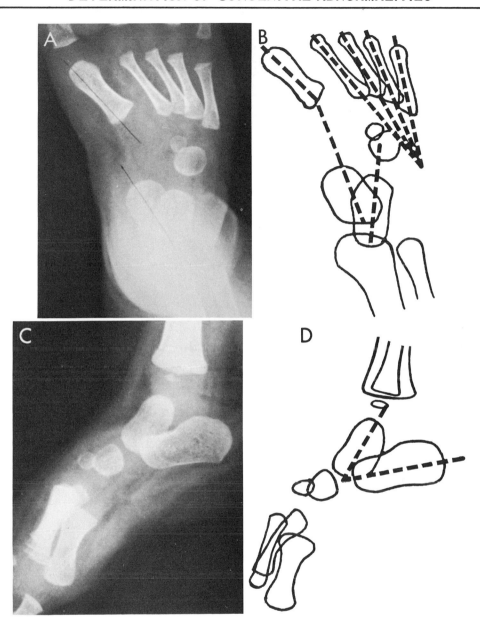

FIG. 157.—Metatarsus varus. *A* and *B*, anteroposterior projection. (1) There is an increased angle between the midtalar line and the line of the shaft of the 1st metatarsal. (2) The lines of the metatarsals converge posteriorly. (3) The midcalcaneal line runs lateral to the normal position. *C* and *D*, lateral projection. (1) The angle between the midcalcaneal and midtalar line may increase. (From Davis and Hatt, Fig. 6.)

169

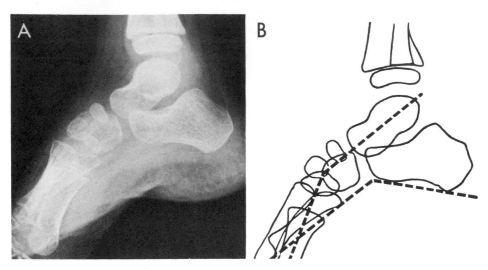

FIG. 158.—Pes cavus. The anteroposterior projection is unchanged from the normal. *A* and *B*, lateral projection. (1) Increased angle between the line through the inferior cortex of the calcaneus and inferior cortex of the 5th metatarsal. (2) There is now an angle between the midtalar line and the line through the shaft of the 1st metatarsal. (From Davis and Hatt, Fig. 7.)

1. *Technique*

   a) Central ray: Perpendicular to plane of film, over midportion of foot in both projections.

   b) Position: Anteroposterior and lateral. Technique must be carefully standardized. *Slight variations in rotation in either projection can markedly alter the relationship of the bones, as shown on the film.* For the anteroposterior view, the knees must be held together and must fall in a plane which is perpendicular to the film (Fig. 152, *A*). The tendency of the technician to "correct" the abnormality by placing the foot normally on the cassette must be discouraged. For the lateral projection (Fig. 152, *B*), the technique for a lateral ankle view is the correct one. Templeton and his co-workers exert pressure against the foot with a plastic board in both projections, to simulate weight bearing.

   c) Target-film distance: Immaterial.

2. *Measurements*

   Figure 153: Normal foot. Recorded angles with weight bearing.
   Figure 154: Clubfoot.
   Figure 155: "Rocker" deformity.
   Figure 156: Flatfoot.
   Figure 157: Metatarsus varus.
   Figure 158: Pes cavus.

3. *Source of Material*

   Davis and Hatt's diagrams described here are not based on any statistically valid sample. They are arranged as a guide for the radiologist in describing certain abnormalities. No particular numbers are assigned to the angles, and the context should be interpreted in a manner similar to that for any other descriptive radiologic finding.

   The angles of the normal foot reported by Templeton *et al.* are based on anteroposterior and lateral weight-bearing roentgenograms of 160 normal children, ages 12 days to 12 years.

MEASUREMENT OF THE HEEL PAD AS AN AID TO
DIAGNOSIS OF ACROMEGALY*

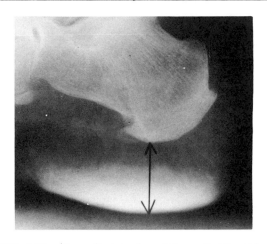

FIG. 159.—(From Steinbach and Russell, Fig. 2.)

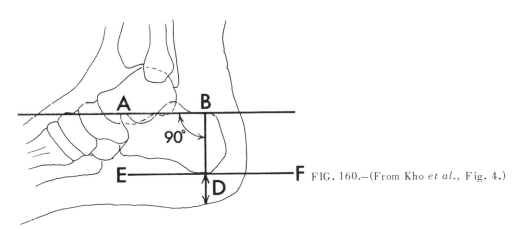

FIG. 160.—(From Kho *et al.*, Fig. 4.)

FIG. 161.—(From Kho *et al.*, Fig. 7.)

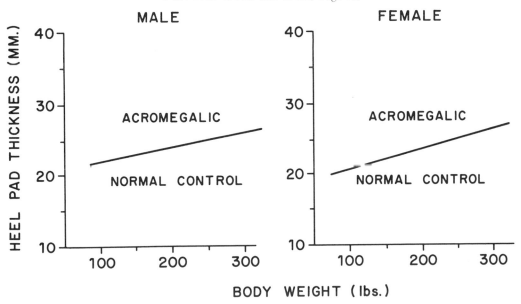

---

*Steinbach, H. L., and Russell, W.: Radiology 82:418, 1964.

MEASUREMENT OF THE HEEL PAD AS AN AID TO
DIAGNOSIS OF ACROMEGALY

1. Technique

a) Central ray: Perpendicular to plane of film centered over the calcaneus.
b) Position: Lateral.
c) Target-film distance: 40 inches.

2. Measurements

See Figures 159 and 160.

The heel pad is measured at the shortest distance between the calcaneus and the plantar surface of the skin. Kho and colleagues* recommend the method shown in Figure 160.

Line *AB* joins the anterior and posterior angles on the superior surface of the calcaneus. Parallel to this line draw line *EF* parallel to the lowest point on the calcaneus. A line perpendicular to this point to the skin surface gives the heel pad thickness *(D)*.

Heel pad thickness is related to body weight (Fig. 161). Puckette and Seymour[†] found a higher mean value in Negroes than in Caucasians and noted that age and sex did not appear to influence heel pad thickness.

HEEL PAD THICKNESS IN CONTROLS*

Mean	S.D.	Upper Limit	
		Male	Female
18.6 mm.	2.6 mm.	25 mm.	23 mm.

3. Source of Material

Steinback and Russell studied 29 patients with unequivocal clinical and laboratory evidence of acromegaly. The control group included 103 normal subjects.

Kho and colleagues studied 79 patients with untreated acromegaly and 52 normal control subjects.

Note:

Several articles have appeared on heel pad thickness.

Most of the articles are listed as references in Kho *et al.*

Two other measurements used less frequently as an aid in the diagnosis of acromegaly are:

a) The Sesamoid Index,[**] which is the product of the two longest perpendicular diameters of the medial sesamoid bone at the metacarpophalangeal joint of the first digit. Median index is 20; range is 12 to 29.
b) Skin thickness.[††] This measurement requires the use of a block of wood to flatten the skin surface. Normal measurements are compared with those found in several types of endocrine disease.

---

*Kho, K. M.; Wright, A. D.; and Doyle, F. H.: Brit. J. Radiol. 43:119, 1970.

[†]Puckette, S. E., and Seymour, E. Q.: Radiology 88:982, 1967.

[**]Kleinberg, D. L.; Young, I. S.; and Kupperman, H. S.: Ann. Int. Med. 64:1075, 1966.

[††]Sheppard, R. H., and Meema, H. E.: Ann. Int. Med. 66:531, 1967.

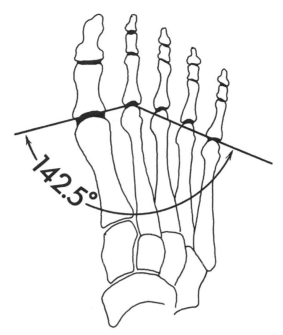

FIG. 162.—(Redrawn from Gamble and Yale, Fig. 199.)

1. *Technique*

    a) Central ray: Perpendicular to plane of film, over midportion of foot.
    b) Position: Anteroposterior.
    c) Target-film distance: Immaterial.

2. *Measurements*

    See Figure 162.
    Total joint line angle 142.5° mean.
    First metatarsal is shorter than second.
    Second metatarsal is longest.
    Third metatarsal is shorter than second.
    Fourth metatarsal is shorter than third.
    Fifth metatarsal is shorter than fourth.

3. *Source of Material*

    Gamble and Yale used 279 foot roentgenograms.

---

*Gamble, F. O., and Yale, I.: *Clinical Foot Roentgenology* (Baltimore: Williams & Wilkins Co., 1966), pp. 158.

IV. THE RESPIRATORY SYSTEM

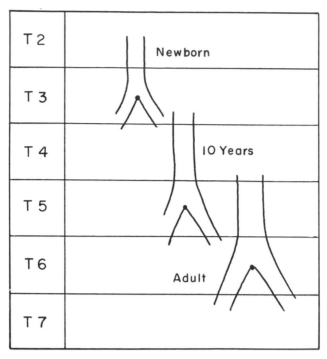

FIG. 163.—Vertebral levels of trachea bifurcation.

1. Technique

    a) Central ray: To 4th thoracic vertebra.

    b) Position: Posteroanterior.

    c) Target-film distance: 72 inches.

2. Measurements

See Figure 163.

Newborn: Third thoracic vertebra.
10 year old: Fifth thoracic vertebra.
Adult: Sixth thoracic vertebra.

3. Source of Material

Caffey quotes the work of Mehnert.[†] The number of cases studied by Mehnert is not known.

*Caffey, J.: *Pediatric X-Ray Diagnosis* (3d ed.; Chicago: Year Book Publishers, Inc., 1956).

†Mehnert, E.: Über topographische Alterveränderungen des Atmungsapparates (Jena, 1901).

MEASUREMENT OF TRACHEA DIAMETER IN THE NEWBORN INFANT*

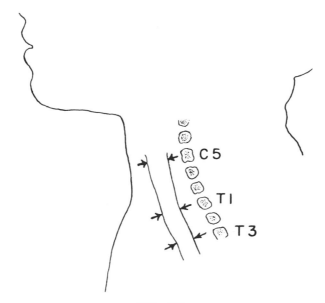

FIG. 164.

1. Technique

    a) Central ray: Anteroposterior—To 4th thoracic vertebra.

                             Left lateral—To 4th thoracic vertebra on midcoronal plane.

    b) Position: Anteroposterior.

                             Left lateral.

    c) Target-film distance: 36 inches.

    Films taken in maximum inspiration.

2. Measurements

See Figure 164.

ANTEROPOSTERIOR DIAMETER OF TRACHEA

Level of measurement	C5	T1	T3
Average diameter (mm.)	4.5	3.9	3.5

LATERAL DIAMETER OF TRACHEA†

Level of measurement	C5	T1	T3
Minimum diameter (mm.)	2	1	1
Maximum diameter (mm.)	7	6	5

    †Donaldson and Tompsett found that this diameter was quite variable. Also, they considered a 3 mm. anteroposterior diameter in the upper thorax to be the lower limit of normal.

3. Source of Material

Studies of 350 normal infants were made within 24 hours after birth.

*Donaldson, S. W., and Tompsett, A. C.: Am. J. Roentgenol. 67:785, 1952.

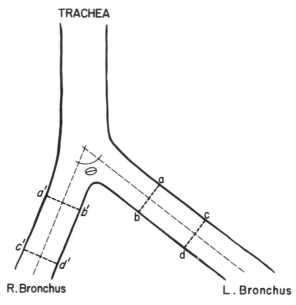

FIG. 165.

1. *Technique*

   a) Central ray: To the 4th thoracic vertebra.
   b) Position: Posteroanterior.
   c) Target-film distance: 40 inches for patients under age 1 year.
       72 inches for all other patients.

2. *Measurements*

   See Figure 165.
       Draw a straight line in the middle of each bronchus parallel to the walls of the bronchus.
       Bifurcation angle *0* is given in Figures 166 and 167. Mean and 95% confidence limits are shown.

*Alavi, S. M.; Keats, T. E.; and O'Brien, W. M.: Am. J. Roentgenol. 108:546, 1970.

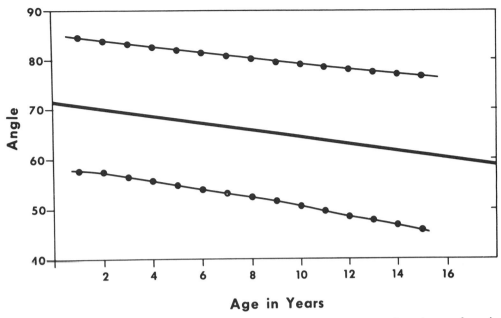

FIG. 166.—95% confidence band for people <16. Regression equation based on male and female data.

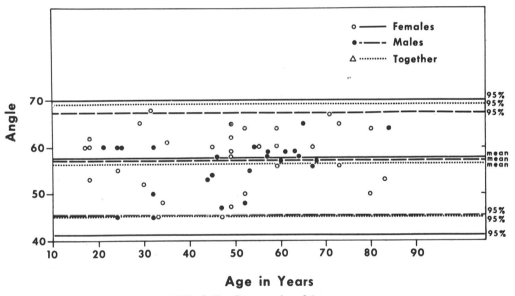

FIG. 167.—Greater than 16 years.

3. *Source of Material*

Eighty-seven patients whose chest roentgenograms were interpreted as normal. Forty-one males and 46 females were in the study. Twenty-nine of the patients were under 16 years of age.

MEASUREMENT OF THE HILUS OUTLINES*

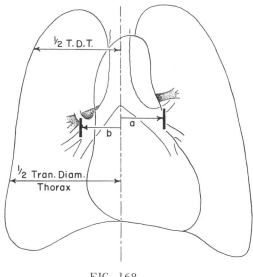

FIG. 168.

1. *Technique*

   a) Central ray: To 4th thoracic vertebral body.

   b) Position: Posteroanterior chest.

   c) Target-film distance: 72 inches.

2. *Measurements*

   See Figure 168.

   Mean width for right and left hili: 5.56 ± 0.12 cm.

   Minimum width, 3.5 cm.

   Maximum width, 7.0 cm.

   Sum of transverse diameters of right and left hili = 11.0 ± 0.03 cm.

   In at least 84% of the cases the difference between the right and left hilus did not exceed 1.0 cm.

   Lateral border of the hilus is the margin farthest from the midline (midline to *b* and to *a* in Figure 168 but not including the first branchings of each pulmonary artery. Rigler and his co-workers found that in 100 patients with proved bronchogenic carcinoma the mean sum of the hili diameters was 13 cm. If either hilus is over 7.0 cm. or if the sum of the diameters is 13 cm., the chance of abnormality is about 90%.

   However, Lodwick, Keats, and Dorst,[†] in a study of 541 cases of proved bronchogenic carcinoma, found that only 31.9% of the cases had a total transverse diameter over 13 cm.; only 36.8% of the cases had a unilateral measurement greater than 7.0 cm.; and 13.5% had a total transverse diameter of less than the mean normal diameter of 11 cm.

   In the very early bronchogenic cancer cases, hilar measurements were abnormal in only 19.4% of the cases.

3. *Source of Material*

   Chest roentgenograms of 100 consecutive patients over 40 years of age, made as hospital routine on admission, were studied.

---

*Rigler, L. G.; O'Laughlin, B.J.; and Tucker, R. C.: Radiology 59:683, 1952.

†Lodwick, G.; Keats, T.E.; and Dorst, J.: Radiology 71:370, 1958.

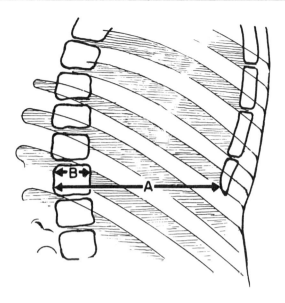

FIG. 169.—(Redrawn from Backer.)

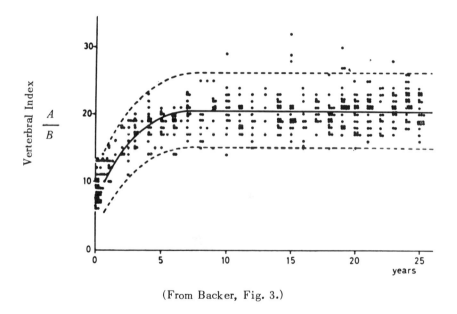

(From Backer, Fig. 3.)

*Backer, O., *et al.:* Acta radiol. 55:249, 1961.

MEASUREMENTS FOR RADIOLOGIC EVALUATION OF FUNNEL CHEST

1. *Technique*

   a) Central ray: Perpendicular to plane of film centered over midchest.
   b) Position: True lateral.
   c) Target-film distance: Immaterial.

2. *Measurements*

   See Figure 169.

   The vertebral index indicates the percentage ratio between the minimum sagittal diameter of the chest, measured from the posterior surface of the vertebral body to the nearest point on the body of the sternum *(A)* and the sagittal diameter of the vertebral body at the same level *(B)*. Figure 169 shows the vertebral index in normal persons. The solid line represents the mean curve. The 95% range lies between the broken lines. This method is applicable in assessing the late results of operation, which heretofore have been based on subjective estimation.

3. *Source of Material*

   The data are based on a normal series of 445 subjects — 197 males and 248 females — about equally distributed in 5 year age groups from 0 to 25 years.

MEASUREMENT OF THE STRAIGHT-BACK SYNDROME*

Absence of the normal thoracic kyphosis is a recently accepted cause of "pseudo heart disease." Roentgenographically, the heart is usually normal in size and configuration, but in some cases it is "pancake" in appearance and in other patients it is displaced to the left with prominence of the pulmonary arteries.

1. *Technique*

   a) Central ray: PA chest: to 4th thoracic vertebral body.
   　　　　　　　　Lateral chest: centered over midchest
   b) Position: Posteroanterior and true lateral
   c) Target-film distance: Posteroanterior: 72 inches
   　　　　　　　　　　　　Lateral: 72 inches

2. *Measurements*

   24 patients with Straight-Back Syndrome

	A-P Chest Diam. (cm.)	*A-P/Transthoracic* Ratio (%)
Males (12)	10.6	35.8
Females (12)	9.8	37.3
100 normal patients		
Males (50)	14.2	47.0
Females (50)	12.0	45.7

3. *Source of Material*

   Twenty-four men and women in whom loss of thoracic kyphosis was the only somatic fault.

---

*Twigg, H. L., *et al.*: Radiology 88:274, 1967.

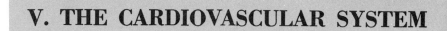

V. THE CARDIOVASCULAR SYSTEM

MEASUREMENT OF THE HEART IN CHILDREN

A. Cardiothoracic Index

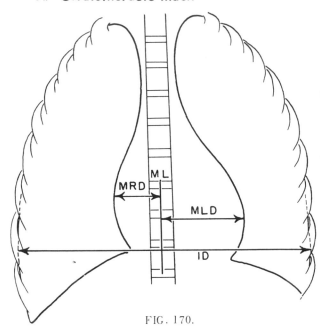

FIG. 170.

FIRST YEAR OF LIFE*

AGE RANGE IN WEEKS	NO. OF CASES	MEAN CARDIO-THORACIC INDEX	RANGE INCLUDED WITHIN 1 S.D.
0- 3	52	0.55	0.60-0.50
4- 7	36	0.58	0.64-0.52
8-15	71	0.57	0.62-0.51
16-23	42	0.57	0.62-0.51
24-31	27	0.56	0.61-0.50
32-39	35	0.56	0.61-0.51
40-47	19	0.54	0.60-0.49
48-55	22	0.53	0.57-0.49

FIRST 6 YEARS OF LIFE[†]

AGE IN YEARS	NO. OF CASES	MEAN CARDIO-THORACIC INDEX	ACTUAL TOTAL RANGE
0-1	357	0.49	0.65-0.39
1-2	211	0.49	0.60-0.39
2-3	183	0.45	0.50-0.39
3-4	152	0.45	0.52-0.40
4-5	87	0.45	0.52-0.40
5-6	33	0.45	0.50-0.40

7-12 YEARS[‡]

AGE IN YEARS	NO. OF CASES	TOTAL TRANSVERSE DIAMETER OF HEART, IN CM.	INTERNAL DIAMETER OF THORAX, IN CM.	NORMAL RANGE
BOYS				
7	35	9.2	19.7	0.49-0.43
8	32	9.4	20.5	0.49-0.42
9	35	9.5	21.1	0.49-0.41
10	21	9.8	21.5	0.49-0.43
11	21	9.9	22.0	0.49-0.43
12	19	10.1	23.0	0.46-0.40
GIRLS				
7	36	9.1	19.3	0.50-0.44
8	32	9.3	20.0	0.50-0.44
9	28	9.5	20.6	0.49-0.43
10	22	9.7	20.9	0.49-0.43
11	24	9.9	22.0	0.49-0.41
12	21	10.4	22.9	0.49-0.41

*Bakwin, H., and Bakwin, R. M.: Am. J. Dis. Child. 49:861, 1935.

[†]Maresh, M. M., and Washburn, A. H.: Am. J. Dis. Child. 56:33, 1938.

[‡]Lincoln, E. M., and Spillman, R.: Am. J. Dis. Child. 35:791, 1928.

(The three tables shown above are arranged as in Caffey, J.: *Pediatric X-Ray Diagnosis* [2d ed.; Chicago: Year Book Publishers, Inc., 1945].)

MEASUREMENT OF THE HEART IN CHILDREN

A. Cardiothoracic Index

1. Technique

a) Central ray: Perpendicular to plane of film centered over midpoint of chest.

b) Positions: Bakwin and Bakwin—Anteroposterior erect. No timing according to phase of respiration.

           Maresh and Washburn—Infants, posteroanterior supine; from age 3 or 3½ years, posteroanterior erect.

           Lincoln and Spillman—Posteroanterior erect. Moderately deep inspiration.

c) Target-film distance: Bakwin and Bakwin—2 meters.

           Maresh and Washburn—Infants, 1.5 meters (5 feet); from 3 or 3½ years, 2.1 meters (7 feet).

           Lincoln and Spillman—6 feet.

2. Measurements

See Figure 170 and tables accompanying figure.

MRD = Maximum transverse diameter of the right side of the heart, which is a line drawn from the midline of the spine to the most distant point on the right cardiac margin.

MLD = Maximum transverse diameter on the left side of the heart.

ID   = Internal diameter of the thorax drawn parallel to the transverse cardiac diameters through the tip of the dome of the right side of the diaphragm. It extends from the right to the left pleural surface.

The total transverse cardiac diameter is the sum of MRD and MLD (MRD and MLD are maximum heart widths to right and left, respectively, of midthoracic line). The cardiothoracic index is obtained by dividing the sum of MRD and MLD by ID. Originally, the heart was considered to be pathologically enlarged when the ratio exceeded 0.50. Experience has demonstrated that there is a considerable range for the normal values of the cardiothoracic index, the range being widest during the first year of life.

3. Source of Material

Bakwin and Bakwin: Data based on study of 165 infant boys and 146 infant girls born in Bellevue Hospital. Only infants of Caucasian antecedents were studied.

Maresh and Washburn: Data based on study of 38 normal boys and 29 normal girls examined by the Child Research Council every 3 months since birth. A total of 1,026 roentgenograms were measured.

Lincoln and Spillman: Study made over a period of 7 school years and based on yearly roentgenograms of 246 normal school children.

B. Transverse Cardiac Diameter
Ages between 4 and 16 years.

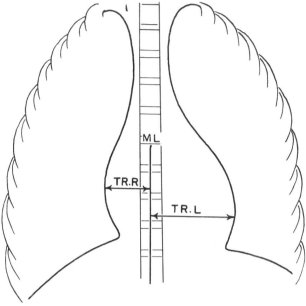

FIG. 171.

TABLE FOR DETERMINING PER CENT DEVIATION FROM AVERAGE *

% MINUS —					AV'GE	% PLUS +				
25	20	15	10	5	%	5	10	15	20	25
51	55	58	62	65	**69**	72	76	79	83	86
52	56	59	63	66	**70**	73	77	80	84	87
52	56	59	63	67	**71**	75	79	83	86	90
53	57	61	64	68	**72**	76	80	83	87	91
54	58	62	65	69	**73**	77	81	84	88	92
55	59	63	66	70	**74**	78	82	85	89	93
57	60	64	68	71	**75**	79	82	86	90	94
58	61	64	68	72	**76**	80	84	88	91	95
59	62	65	69	73	**77**	81	85	89	92	96
59	62	66	70	74	**78**	82	86	90	94	98
60	63	67	71	75	**79**	83	87	91	95	99
61	64	68	72	76	**80**	84	88	92	96	100
62	65	69	73	77	**81**	85	89	93	97	101
63	66	70	74	78	**82**	86	90	94	98	102
63	66	71	75	78	**83**	87	91	95	100	104
64	67	71	76	80	**84**	88	92	97	101	105
65	68	72	76	81	**85**	89	94	98	102	106
66	69	73	77	82	**86**	90	95	99	103	107
67	70	74	78	83	**87**	91	96	100	104	108
67	70	75	79	84	**88**	92	97	101	106	110
68	72	76	80	85	**89**	93	98	102	107	111
69	72	76	81	86	**90**	94	99	104	108	112
70	73	77	82	86	**91**	96	100	105	109	113
71	74	78	83	87	**92**	97	101	106	110	114
71	74	79	84	88	**93**	98	102	107	112	117
72	75	80	85	89	**94**	99	103	108	113	118
72	76	81	85	90	**95**	100	105	109	114	119
73	77	82	86	91	**96**	101	106	110	115	120
74	78	82	87	92	**97**	102	107	112	116	120
74	78	83	88	93	**98**	103	108	113	118	123
75	79	84	89	94	**99**	104	109	114	119	124
75	80	85	90	95	**100**	105	110	115	120	125
76	81	86	91	96	**101**	106	111	116	121	126
77	82	87	92	97	**102**	107	112	117	122	127
78	82	88	93	98	**103**	108	113	118	124	129
79	83	88	94	99	**104**	109	114	120	125	130
80	84	89	95	100	**105**	110	116	121	126	131
81	85	90	95	101	**106**	111	117	122	127	132
82	86	91	96	102	**107**	112	118	123	128	133
82	86	92	97	103	**108**	113	119	124	130	135
83	87	93	98	104	**109**	114	120	125	131	136
84	88	94	99	105	**110**	116	121	127	132	137
85	89	94	100	105	**111**	117	122	128	133	138
85	90	95	101	106	**112**	118	123	129	134	139
85	90	96	102	107	**113**	119	124	130	136	141
86	91	97	103	108	**114**	120	125	131	137	142
87	92	98	104	109	**115**	121	127	132	138	143
88	93	99	104	110	**116**	122	128	133	139	144
89	94	99	105	111	**117**	123	129	135	140	145
89	94	100	106	112	**118**	124	130	136	142	147
90	95	101	107	113	**119**	125	131	137	143	149
91	96	102	108	114	**120**	126	132	138	144	150
92	97	103	109	115	**121**	127	133	139	145	151
93	98	104	110	116	**122**	128	134	140	146	152
93	98	105	111	117	**123**	129	135	141	148	153
94	99	105	112	118	**124**	130	136	143	149	155
95	100	106	113	119	**125**	131	138	144	150	156
96	101	107	113	120	**126**	132	139	145	151	157
97	102	108	114	121	**127**	133	140	146	152	158
97	102	109	115	122	**128**	134	141	147	154	160
98	103	110	116	123	**129**	135	142	148	155	161
99	104	111	117	124	**130**	137	143	150	156	162
100	105	111	118	124	**131**	138	144	151	157	163
101	106	112	119	125	**132**	139	145	152	158	164

*From Esguerra-Gomez, G. E.: Bol. clinica de Marly, Vol. 11, Nos. 5-8, 1949.

MEASUREMENT OF THE HEART IN CHILDREN

B. Transverse Cardiac Diameter

TABLE FOR PREDICTION OF TRANSVERSE CARDIAC DIAMETER IN CHILDREN *

$$D \text{ (in cms)} = 2\sqrt{\dfrac{\text{Weight (in kilos)}}{\text{Height (in meters)}}}$$

IN.	CM.	14	15	16	17	18	19	20	21	22	23	24	25	26	27	28	29	30	31	32	33	34	35	36	37	38	39	40	41
30	76	86	89																										
	77	86	89																										
31	78	85	88	91																									
	79	85	88	91																									
	80	84	87	90																									
32	81	84	87	90	92																								
	82	83	86	89	92																								
	83	83	86	89	91																								
33	84	82	85	88	91	93																							
	85	82	85	88	90	93																							
34	86	81	84	87	90	92																							
	87	81	84	86	89	92	94																						
	88	80	83	86	89	91	93																						
35	89	80	83	85	88	91	93																						
	90	79	82	85	88	90	92	95																					
36	91	79	82	84	87	90	92	94																					
	92	79	81	84	87	89	91	94																					
	93	78	81	83	86	89	91	93	96																				
37	94	78	80	83	86	88	90	93	95																				
	95	77	80	82	85	88	90	92	95																				
38	96	77	80	82	85	87	89	92	94	96																			
	97	76	79	82	84	87	89	91	94	96																			
39	98	76	79	81	84	86	88	91	93	95																			
	99	76	78	81	83	86	88	90	93	95	97																		
	100	75	78	81	83	85	88	90	92	94	96																		
40	101	75	77	80	82	85	87	89	92	94	96																		
	102	74	77	80	82	84	87	89	91	93	95	98																	
	103	74	77	79	82	84	86	88	91	93	95	97																	
41	104	74	76	79	81	84	86	88	90	92	94	97																	
	105	73	76	78	81	83	86	88	90	92	94	96	98																
42	106	73	76	78	80	83	85	87	89	91	93	96	98																
	107	73	75	78	80	82	85	87	89	91	93	95	97																
	108	72	75	77	80	82	84	86	88	91	92	95	97	99															
43	109	73	75	77	79	82	84	86	88	90	92	94	96	98															
	110	72	74	77	79	81	83	86	88	90	92	94	96	98															
44	111	71	74	76	79	81	83	85	87	89	91	93	95	97	99														
	112	71	74	76	78	80	83	85	87	89	91	93	95	97	99														
	113	71	73	76	78	80	82	84	86	89	91	92	94	96	98														
45	114	70	73	75	78	80	82	84	86	88	90	92	94	96	98	99													
	115	70	73	75	77	79	82	84	86	88	89	92	94	96	97	99													
46	116	70	72	75	77	79	81	83	85	87	89	91	93	95	97	99													
	117	70	72	74	77	79	81	83	85	87	89	91	93	95	96	98	100												
	118	69	72	74	76	78	81	83	85	87	88	90	92	94	96	98	99												
47	119	69	71	74	76	78	80	82	84	86	88	90	92	94	96	97	99												
	120	69	71	73	76	78	80	82	84	86	88	90	92	94	95	97	99	100											
48	121		71	73	75	77	79	82	84	86	87	89	91	93	95	97	98	100											
	122		70	73	75	77	79	81	83	85	87	89	91	93	95	96	98	100											
	123		70	72	75	77	79	81	83	85	87	89	91	92	94	96	98	99	101										
49	124		70	72	74	76	79	81	82	84	86	88	90	92	94	95	97	99	101										
	125			72	74	76	78	80	82	84	86	88	90	92	93	95	97	98	100										
50	126			72	74	76	78	80	82	84	86	87	89	91	93	95	96	98	100	102									
	127				73	76	78	80	82	83	85	87	89	91	93	94	96	98	100	101									
	128					75	77	79	81	83	85	87	89	90	92	94	96	97	99	101									
51	129					75	77	79	81	83	85	86	88	90	92	94	95	97	99	101	102								
	130						77	79	81	82	84	86	88	90	92	93	95	96	98	100	102	102	104	105	107	108	110	111	112
52	131						76	78	80	82	84	86	88	89	91	93	94	96	98	100	101	102	104	105	106	108	109	110	112
	132						76	78	80	82	84	85	87	89	91	93	94	96	98	99	101	102	103	105	106	107	109	110	111
53	133						76	78	80	82	83	85	87	89	90	92	94	95	97	99	101	102	104	104	106	107	108	110	111
	134								79	81	83	85	87	88	90	92	93	95	97	98	100	101	103	104	105	107	108	109	111
	135									79	81	84	86	88	90	91	93	95	97	98	100	101	102	104	105	106	108	109	110
54	136									81	82	84	86	88	89	91	93	94	96	98	99	101	102	103	105	106	107	108	110
	137									80	82	84	86	87	89	91	92	94	96	97	99	100	102	103	104	106	107	108	109
	138										82	84	85	87	89	90	92	94	96	97	98	100	101	103	104	105	107	108	109
55	139										82	83	85	87	88	90	92	93	95	97	98	99	101	102	104	105	106	107	109
	140											83	85	86	88	90	91	93	95	96	98	99	101	102	103	105	106	107	108
56	141												84	86	88	89	91	92	95	96	97	99	100	102	103	104	106	107	108
	142												84	86	87	89	91	92	94	96	97	98	100	101	103	104	105	106	108
	143														87	88	90	92	94	95	97	98	100	101	102	104	105	106	107
57	144														87	88	90	92	93	95	96	98	99	101	102	103	105	105	107
	145															88	90	91	93	95	96	97	99	100	102	103	104	105	107
58	146															88	89	91	93	94	96	97	99	100	101	103	104	105	106
	147																89	91	92	94	95	97	98	100	101	102	104	105	106
	148																89	90	92	94	95	96	98	99	101	102	103	104	106
59	149																88	90	92	93	95	96	98	99	100	102	103	104	105
	150																88	90	92	93	94	96	97	99	100	101	103		
	151																		91	93	94	95	97	98	100	101	102		
60	152																		91	92	94	95	97	98	99	101	102		

*From Esguerra-Gomez, G.: Bol. clinica de Marly, Vol. II, Nos. 5-8, 1949.

B. Transverse Cardiac Diameter

NOMOGRAM FOR PREDICTION OF TRANSVERSE DIAMETER
IN CHILDREN

$$D(cm) = 2\sqrt{W(kilos)/H(meters)}$$

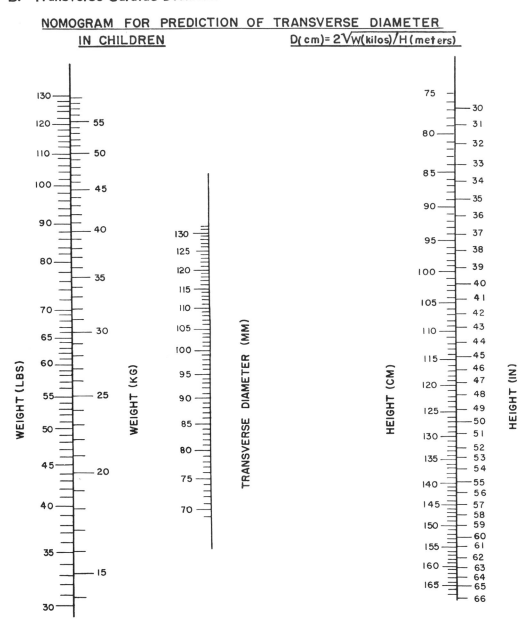

FIG. 172.—(Adapted from Esguerra-Gomez, G. E.: Radiology 57:217, 1951.)

B. Transverse Cardiac Diameter

1. *Technique*

a) Central ray: Perpendicular to plane of film centered over midchest.
b) Position: Erect, posteroanterior. Moderate inspiration.
c) Target-film distance: At least 6 feet.

2. *Measurements*

See Figure 171.

ML = Midline.
$TR.R$ = Maximum transverse cardiac diameter, right.
$TR.L$ = Maximum transverse cardiac diameter, left.
Transverse cardiac diameter equals $TR.R$ plus $TR.L$.

These measurements are based on measured length of the transverse cardiac diameter in relation to the anthropometric index. In children between 9 and 16 years of age, the mean values show an insignificant negative deviation that probably coincides with accumulation of fat in subcutaneous tissues during growth periods.

A constant to establish a predicted cardiac transverse diameter in children was determined. The constant is:

$$\frac{\text{Weight (kg.)} \times 100,000}{\text{Height (cm.)} \times (\text{Transverse diameter})^2} = 2.47$$

With the aid of this constant, prediction tables and a nomogram were made (see Fig. 172). Analyzing the studies of Maresh* in relation to the prediction tables, the anthropometric indices, and the average of weights and heights, it is found that the cardiac measurements of 81.2% of the examined children between the ages of 4 and 16 years fall between +10 and −10 per cent of the prediction tables. Between the ages of 4 and 8 years, the percentage is 88.53%.

These records studied on the respective histograms establish that there exists a relationship between the transverse diameter of the heart and the anthropometric index, not only in adults but in children as well. From 4 to 8 years of age, the histogram coincides with that of adults, and we explain the slight minus deviation from 9 to 15 years of age as the result of the subcutaneous accumulation of fat during growth periods.

3. *Source of Material*

The data are based on a study by Maresh. In her study a group of 71 boys and 57 girls were examined radiologically several times a year over a period of more than 20 years. Of a total of 3,205 roentgenograms, only 3,190 gave the necessary data (transverse diameter of the heart, weight, and height). The data of Gomez are based exclusively on this group.

---

*Maresh, M. M.: Pediatrics 2:382, 1948.

A. The Cardiothoracic Ratio*

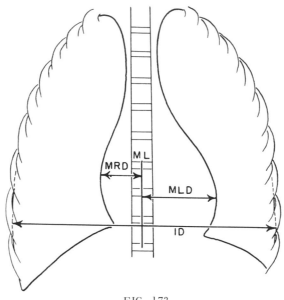

FIG. 173.

*Danzer, C. S.: Am. J. M. Sc. 157:513, 1919.

MEASUREMENT OF THE HEART AND AORTA IN ADULTS

A. The Cardiothoracic Ratio

1. *Technique*

a) Central ray: Perpendicular to plane of film centered over midportion of chest.
b) Position: Posteroanterior erect. Breathing suspended in midrespiration.
c) Target-film distance: 6 feet.

2. *Measurements*

See Figure 173.

MRD = Maximum transverse diameter of the right side of the heart, which is a line drawn from the midline of the spine to the most distant point on the right cardiac margin.

ML = Midline of the spine.

MLD = Maximum transverse diameter on the left side of the heart.

ID = Greatest internal diameter of the thorax, which is usually at the level of the apex or one space lower, measuring the inner borders of the ribs.

The transverse diameter *(TD)* of the heart = MRD + MLD.

The cardiothoracic ratio

$$= \frac{\text{Maximum transverse diameter heart } (TD)}{\text{Maximum transverse diameter thorax } (ID)}$$

The normal heart is usually less than half the greatest diameter of the thorax. The normal cardiothoracic ratio varies between 39% and 50%, with an average of about 45%. Because of variations due to cardiac filling and phase of respiration, a margin of safety of 2% above the upper limit is claimed.

3. *Source of Material*

The method was tested on approximately 500 patients. In Danzer's opinion, the results of this test warrant its practicability and usefulness in the estimation of cardiac size, particularly in cases of moderate or early enlargement.

4. *Cardiac Measurements in Systole and Diastole*[*]

a) Two chest films obtained on each of 359 patients.
b) Films taken during systole and diastole.
c) Summary of size changes in the widest transverse measurements of the heart.

Differences in Heart Size	No. of Patients	Percent of Patients
0.0 to 0.3 cm.	169	52
0.4 to 0.9 cm.	113	41
1.0 to 1.7 cm.	22	7

---

[*]Gammill, S. L.; Krebs, C.; Meyers, P.; *et al.:* Radiology 94:115, 1970.

B. The Ungerleider Method*

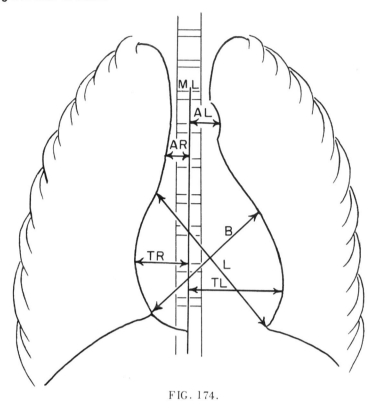

FIG. 174.

*Ungerleider, H. E., and Gubner, R.: Am. Heart J. 24:494, 1942.

MEASUREMENT OF THE HEART AND AORTA IN ADULTS

B. The Ungerleider Method

THEORETICAL TRANSVERSE DIAMETERS OF HEART AND AORTIC SILHOUETTE FOR VARIOUS HEIGHTS AND WEIGHTS*

TABLE FOR DETERMINING PERCENT DEVIATION FROM AVERAGE*

AORTA T.D. MM	HEART T.D. MM	HEIGHT 5'0"	1"	2"	3"	4"	5"	6"	7"	8"	9"	10"	11"	6'0"	1"	2"	3"	4"	5"	6"	% MINUS — 25	20	15	10	5	▼	% PLUS + 5	10	15	20	25
47	100	83	85	86	87	89	90	92													75	80	85	90	95	100	105	110	115	120	125
	101	85	86	88	89	91	92	93	95												76	81	86	91	96	101	106	111	116	121	126
	102	87	88	90	91	92	94	95	97			LIGHT FIGURES REPRESENT WEIGHTS									77	82	87	92	97	102	107	112	117	122	128
	103	88	90	92	93	94	96	97	99	100											77	82	88	93	98	103	108	113	118	124	129
	104	90	92	93	95	96	98	99	101	102											78	83	88	94	99	104	109	114	120	125	130
49	105	92	93	95	96	98	99	101	103	104	106										79	84	89	95	100	105	110	116	121	126	131
	106	94	95	97	98	100	101	103	104	106	108										80	85	90	95	101	106	111	117	122	127	133
	107	95	97	99	100	102	103	105	106	108	110	111									80	86	91	96	102	107	112	118	123	128	134
	108	97	99	100	102	104	105	107	108	110	112	113									81	86	92	97	103	108	113	119	124	130	135
	109	99	101	102	104	106	107	109	110	112	114	115	117								82	87	93	98	104	109	114	120	125	131	136
52	110	101	102	104	106	108	109	111	113	114	116	118	119	121							83	88	94	99	105	110	116	121	127	132	138
	111	103	104	106	108	109	111	113	115	116	118	120	121	123	125						83	89	94	100	105	111	117	122	128	133	139
	112	105	106	108	110	111	113	115	117	118	120	122	124	125	127	129					84	90	95	101	106	112	118	123	129	134	140
	113	106	108	110	112	113	115	117	119	121	123	124	126	128	129	131	133				85	90	96	102	107	113	119	124	130	136	141
	114	108	110	112	114	115	117	119	121	123	125	126	128	130	132	133	135	137			86	91	97	103	108	114	120	125	131	137	143
54	115	110	112	114	116	117	119	121	123	125	127	129	130	132	134	136	138	140	141		86	92	98	104	109	115	121	127	132	138	144
	116	112	114	116	118	120	121	123	125	127	129	131	133	134	136	138	140	142	144	146	87	93	99	104	110	116	122	128	133	139	145
	117	114	116	118	120	122	124	125	127	129	131	133	135	137	139	141	143	144	146	148	88	94	99	105	111	117	123	129	135	140	146
	118	116	118	120	122	124	126	128	129	131	133	135	137	139	141	143	145	147	149	151	89	94	100	106	112	118	124	130	136	142	148
	119	118	120	122	124	126	128	130	132	134	136	138	140	142	143	145	147	149	151	153	89	95	101	107	113	119	125	131	137	143	149
56	120	120	122	124	126	128	130	132	134	136	138	140	142	144	146	148	150	152	154	156	90	96	102	108	114	120	126	132	138	144	150
	121	122	124	126	128	130	132	134	136	138	140	142	144	146	148	150	152	154	156	159	91	97	103	109	115	121	127	133	139	145	151
	122	124	126	128	130	132	134	136	138	140	143	145	147	149	151	153	155	157	159	161	92	98	104	110	116	122	128	134	140	146	152
	123	126	128	130	132	134	136	139	141	143	145	147	149	151	153	155	157	160	162	164	92	98	105	111	117	123	129	135	141	148	154
	124	128	130	132	134	137	139	141	143	145	147	149	152	154	156	158	160	162	164	166	93	99	105	112	118	124	130	136	143	149	155
58	125	130	132	134	137	139	141	143	145	147	150	152	154	156	158	160	163	165	167	169	94	100	106	113	119	125	131	138	144	150	156
	126	132	134	137	139	141	143	145	148	150	152	154	156	159	161	163	165	167	170	172	95	101	107	113	120	126	132	139	145	151	158
	127	134	137	139	141	143	146	148	150	152	154	157	159	161	163	166	168	170	172	175	95	102	108	114	121	127	133	140	146	152	159
	128	136	139	141	143	146	148	150	152	155	157	159	161	164	166	168	171	173	175	177	96	102	109	115	122	128	134	141	147	154	160
	129	139	141	143	146	148	150	152	155	157	159	162	164	166	169	171	173	176	178	180	97	103	110	116	123	129	135	142	148	155	161
61	130	141	143	145	148	150	152	155	157	160	162	164	167	169	171	174	176	178	181	183	98	104	111	117	124	130	137	143	150	156	163
	131	143	145	148	150	152	155	157	160	162	164	167	169	172	174	176	179	181	183	186	98	105	111	118	124	131	138	144	151	157	164
	132	145	148	150	152	155	157	160	162	164	167	169	172	174	177	179	181	184	186	189	99	106	112	119	125	132	139	145	152	158	165
	133	147	150	152	153	[illegible]	[illegible]	[illegible]	[illegible]	[illegible]	[illegible]	[illegible]	[illegible]	[illegible]	[illegible]	[illegible]	[illegible]	[illegible]	[illegible]	[illegible]	100	106	113	120	126	133	140	146	153	160	166
	134	150	152	155	157	160	162	164	167	169	172	174	177	179	182	184	187	189	192	194	101	107	114	121	127	134	141	147	154	161	168
63	135	152	154	157	159	162	164	167	169	172	175	177	180	182	185	187	190	192	195	197	101	108	115	122	128	135	142	149	155	162	169
	136	154	157	159	162	164	167	169	172	175	177	180	182	185	187	190	193	195	198	200	102	109	116	122	129	136	143	150	156	163	170
	137	156	159	162	164	167	169	172	175	177	180	182	185	188	190	193	195	198	201	203	103	110	116	123	130	137	144	151	158	164	171
	138	159	161	164	167	169	172	174	177	180	182	185	188	190	193	196	198	201	204	206	104	110	117	124	131	138	145	152	159	166	173
	139	161	164	166	169	172	174	177	180	182	185	188	190	193	196	198	201	204	206	209	104	111	118	125	132	139	146	153	160	167	174
65	140	163	166	169	171	174	177	180	182	185	188	190	193	196	199	201	204	207	209	212	105	112	119	126	133	140	147	154	161	168	175
	141	166	168	171	174	177	179	182	185	188	190	193	196	199	201	204	207	210	212	215	106	113	120	127	134	141	148	155	162	169	176
	142	168	171	174	176	179	182	185	188	190	193	196	199	202	204	207	210	213	216	218	107	114	121	128	135	142	149	156	163	170	178
	143	170	173	176	179	182	184	187	190	193	196	199	202	204	207	210	213	216	219	221	107	114	122	129	136	143	150	157	164	172	179
	144	173	176	178	181	184	187	190	193	196	199	201	204	207	210	213	216	219	222	224	108	115	122	130	137	144	151	158	166	173	180
67	145	175	178	181	184	187	190	193	196	198	201	204	207	210	213	216	219	222	225	228	109	116	123	131	138	145	152	160	167	174	181
	146	178	180	183	186	189	192	195	198	201	204	207	210	213	216	219	222	225	228	231	110	117	124	131	139	146	153	161	168	175	183
	147	180	183	186	189	192	195	198	201	204	207	210	213	216	219	222	225	228	231	234	110	118	125	132	140	147	154	162	169	176	184
	148	182	185	188	192	195	198	201	204	207	210	213	216	219	222	225	228	231	234	237	111	118	126	133	141	148	155	163	170	178	185
	149	185	188	191	194	197	200	203	206	210	213	216	219	222	225	228	231	234	237	240	112	119	127	134	142	149	156	164	171	179	186
70	150	187	191	194	197	200	203	206	209	212	215	219	222	225	228	231	234	237	240	243	113	120	128	135	143	150	158	165	173	180	188
	151	190	193	196	199	203	206	209	212	215	218	222	225	228	231	234	237	241	244	247	113	121	128	136	143	151	159	166	174	181	189
	152	192	196	199	202	205	208	212	215	218	221	224	228	231	234	237	241	244	247	250	114	122	129	137	144	152	160	167	175	182	190
	153	195	198	201	205	208	211	214	218	221	224	227	231	234	237	240	244	247	250	253	115	122	130	138	145	153	161	168	176	184	191
	154	198	201	204	207	211	214	217	221	224	227	230	234	237	240	244	247	250	253	257	116	123	131	139	146	154	162	169	177	185	193
73	155	200	203	207	210	213	217	220	224	227	230	233	237	240	243	247	250	253	257	260	116	124	132	140	147	155	163	171	178	186	194
	156		206	210	213	216	220	223	227	230	233	236	240	243	247	250	254	257	260	264	117	125	133	140	148	156	164	172	179	187	195
	157				216	219	222	226	229	233	236	239	243	246	250	253	257	260	263	267	118	126	133	141	149	157	165	173	181	188	196
	158						225	229	232	236	239	243	246	249	253	256	260	263	267	270	119	126	134	142	150	158	166	174	182	190	198
	159								235	239	242	246	249	253	256	260	263	267	270	279	119	127	135	143	151	159	167	175	183	191	199
75	160										245	249	252	256	259	263	266	270	274	277	120	128	136	144	152	160	168	176	184	192	200
	161												255	259	263	266	270	273	277	281	121	129	137	145	153	161	169	177	185	193	201
	162												259	262	266	270	273	277	280	284	122	130	138	146	154	162	170	178	186	194	203
	163														269	273	277	280	284	288	122	130	139	147	155	163	171	179	187	196	204
	164														273	276	280	284	287	291	123	131	139	148	156	164	172	180	189	197	205

ACTUAL DIAMETER (mm.) — PREDICTED DIAMETER (mm.) — ACTUAL DIAMETER (mm.)

*Ungerleider, H. E., and Clark, C. P.: Tr. Life Ins. M. Dir. America 25:84, 1938.

B. The Ungerleider Method

NOMOGRAMS FOR AREA AND TRANSVERSE DIAMETER OF FRONTAL HEART SILHOUETTE

A PREDICTED AREA FROM WEIGHT AND HEIGHT, AND ACTUAL AREA FROM LONG AND BROAD DIAMETERS

$$[A = {}^{\pi}/_4 \, L \times B]$$ FOR ORTHODIAGRAM AND TELEOROENTGENOGRAM

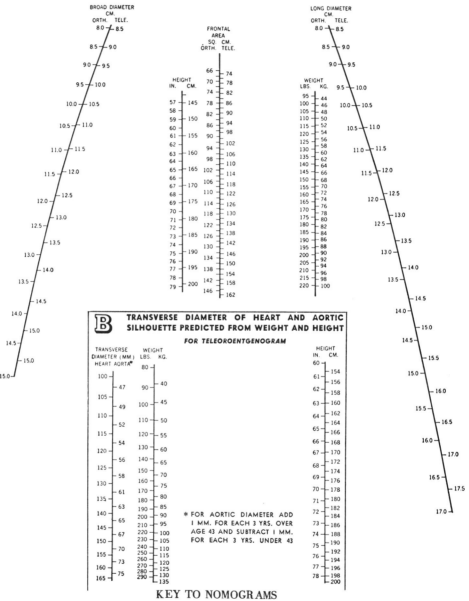

KEY TO NOMOGRAMS

The values for actual (or predicted) area are read at the point at which a straight line extending from the long and broad diameters (or weight and height) intersects the cardiac area scale. Orthodiagram values are on the left, teleoroentgenogram values on the right. In the lower nomogram the predicted transverse diameter of the heart (left side of scale) or aortic arch (right side of scale) is obtained as an extension of a straight line connecting height and weight. A correction for age, as indicated, is necessary for the aortic diameter. Values exceeding 10% above the predicted are abnormal.

FIG. 175.—(From Ungerleider, H. E., and Gubner, R.: Am. Heart J. 24:494 [Fig. 3], 1942.)

MEASUREMENT OF THE HEART AND AORTA IN ADULTS

B. The Ungerleider Method

1. *Technique*

   a) Central ray: Perpendicular to plane of film centered over midchest.

   b) Position: Posteroanterior. Erect or sitting, with respiration suspended at ordinary inspiration.

   c) Target-film distance: 6 feet.

2. *Measurements*

See Figure 174.

   a) For use with tables on page 193.

   TR = Maximum projection to the right heart border from midline.

   TL = Maximum projection to the left heart border from midline.

   TD = Sum of maximum projections to right and left borders from midline
   $= TR + TL$.

   b) For use with nomograms (Fig. 175):

   L = Long diameter. This line extends from the junction of the cardiac and vascular silhouette on the upper part of the right border of the heart obliquely downward to the apex on the left.

   B = Broad diameter. This is the greatest diameter perpendicular to the long diameter. As a rule, it extends from the upper limit of the left ventricular contour to the lowermost point of the right border of the heart. If the heart is transversely placed, it may be necessary to extend the lower right heart border in its natural curve to delineate the margin of the broad diameter.

   c) For use with both tables and nomograms:

   AR = Maximum extension of vascular pedicle to right of midline.

   AL = Maximum extension of vascular pedicle to left of midline.

   Aorta $TD = AR + AL$ = Sum of maximum extensions to right and to left borders of vascular pedicle from midline.

   In the use of the nomogram A, a few simple measurements in relation to standards predicted from weight and height suffice for the estimation of heart size. These are the transverse diameter of the heart and the area of the frontal cardiac silhouette. The latter may be calculated accurately from the product of the long and the broad diameters, which may be conveniently employed in lieu of planimetry. Nomogram A permits the frontal area to be read directly from the long and the broad diameters. Predicted values for the frontal area from weight and height are shown in the same nomogram. In nomogram B are shown the predicted transverse diameters of the heart and of the frontal aortic arch silhouette. An increase in the aortic arch transverse diameter may result from tortuosity as well as from widening of the aorta. Values exceeding 10% above that predicted for frontal area, transverse diameter of the heart, and transverse diameter of the frontal aortic arch are abnormal, since few normal subjects fall outside this range.

3. *Source of Material*

Prediction measurements are based on a study of 1,460 teleoroentgenograms of normal subjects.

ANGIOCARDIOGRAPHIC CIRCULATION TIMES*

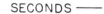

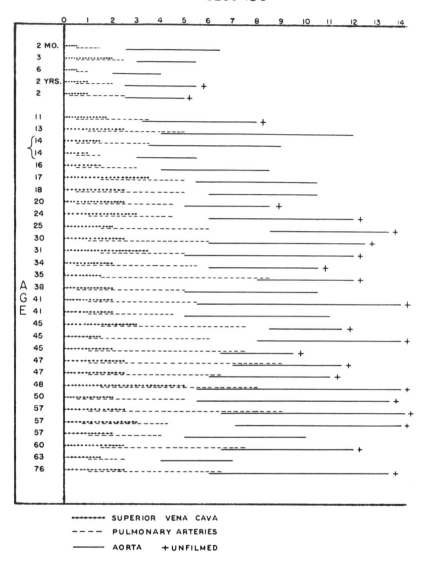

NORMAL OPACIFICATION TIMES

FIG. 176.—Normal opacification periods of the superior vena cava, pulmonary artery and its main branches, and the aorta. Timing begins with the initial entry of the contrast medium into the intrathoracic veins. Note that, with few exceptions, there is no overlapping opacity of the pulmonary arteries and the aorta. (From Figley.)

*Figley, M. M.: Radiology 63:837, 1954.

ANGIOCARDIOGRAPHIC CIRCULATION TIMES

1. Technique

a) Central ray: Perpendicular to plane of film centered over heart.

b) Position: Children up to age 6 or 7 are examined recumbent, with no attempt to control respiration. Older children and adults are examined in a sitting position. Injection is begun with the initiation of a deep but not maximum inspiration, and the breath is held for 12-15 seconds during the entire filming cycle. Dosage was 1 cc. for 2 pounds of weight up to a maximum of 50 cc.

c) Target-film distance: Immaterial.

2. Measurements

See Figure 176.

Circulation times are based on the author's visual estimate of the earliest and latest definite opacification of the structure studied.

3. Source of Material

The data are based on a study of angiocardiograms of 35 patients, most of whom were studied for intrathoracic masses and had no clinical evidence of cardiac disease or compression by the mass. Several others had aneurysms or anomalous aortic branches.

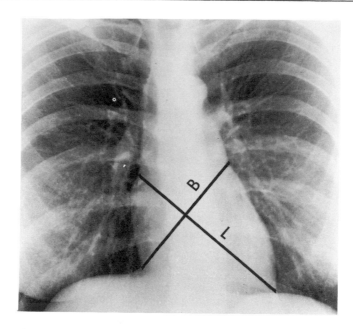

FIG. 177.—(From Keats, T. E., and Enge, I. P.: Radiology 85:850, 1965, Fig. 1.)

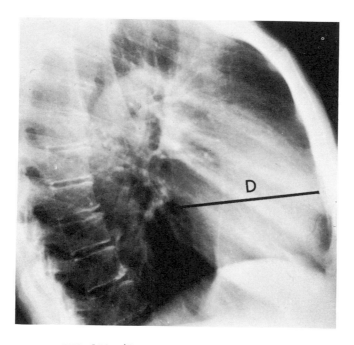

FIG. 178.—(From Keats and Enge, Fig. 1.)

CARDIAC VOLUME IN CHILDREN AND ADOLESCENTS
AS PREDICTED BY BODY WEIGHT*

Body weight (X) in pounds	Cardiac volume (Y) of males (c.c.)			Cardiac volume (Y) of females (c.c.)		
		95% confidence limits			95% confidence limits	
	Mean	Upper limit	Lower limit	Mean	Upper limit	Lower limit
5	27	37	20	29	39	21
10	53	72	40	54	73	39
15	79	107	59	77	105	57
20	104	141	77	101	137	74
25	129	175	95	123	167	91
30	154	209	114	145	197	107
40	204	277	151	189	256	139
50	254	344	187	231	314	170
60	303	411	224	273	370	201
70	352	477	260	314	426	231
80	401	543	296	354	481	261
90	450	610	332	394	535	290
100	498	676	368	434	589	319
110	547	741	404	473	642	348
120	595	807	439	512	695	377
130	644	873	475	550	748	405
140	692	938	510	588	800	433
150	740	1004	545	626	852	461
160	788	1069	580	664	903	489
170	836	1134	616	702	954	516

For males $Y = 5.620 X^{0.973}$ (linear correlation r = 0.982)
For females $Y = 6.628 X^{0.907}$ (linear correlation r = 0.980)

FIG. 179.—(From Nghiem *et al.*, Table 2.)

COMPARISON OF BODY SURFACE AREA AND BODY WEIGHT
AS PREDICTORS OF CARDIAC VOLUME

Sample	No. of Subjects	Correlation Coefficient (r)	Regression Equation	95% Confidence Limits		
				Upper Limit	Lower Limit	% of Mean
Body surface area (Z)						
Limited data	261	0.981	$Y = 284\ Z$	413 Z	155 Z	±45
Males	132	0.980	$= 295\ Z$	434 Z	156 Z	±47
Females	129	0.987	$= 273\ Z$	388 Z	159 Z	±42
Body weight (X)						
Limited data	261	0.987	$Y = 5.0X$	6.6X	3.4X	±32
Males	132	0.990	$= 5.2X$	6.7X	3.7X	±29
Females	129	0.990	$= 4.8X$	6.4X	3.2X	±34
Total data	305	0.985	$Y = 4.9X$	6.6X	3.2X	±34
Males	158	0.985	$Y = 5.1X$	6.8X	3.5X	±32
Females	147	0.989	$Y = 4.7X$	6.3X	3.1X	±34

The limited data included 261 subjects whose height and weight were known. Y = cardiac volume in cubic cm.; X = body weight in pounds; Z = body surface area in square meters.

FIG. 180.—(From Nghiem *et al.*, Table 3.)

---

*Nghiem, Q. X.; Schreiber, M. H.; and Harris, L. C.: Circulation 35:509, 1967.

Nomogram for the Determination
of Body Surface Area of Children

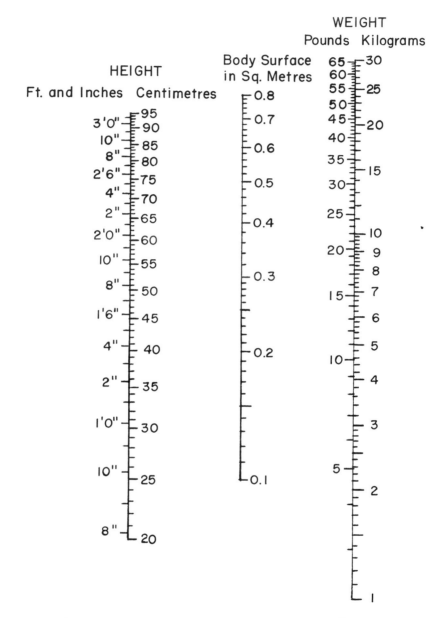

FIG. 181.—(Redrawn from Documenta Geigy, *Scientific Tables* [6th ed.; Basel, Switzerland, 1962].) *(Continued on next page.)*

Predicted Normal Heart Volume Compared with Calculated Heart Volumes in Infants

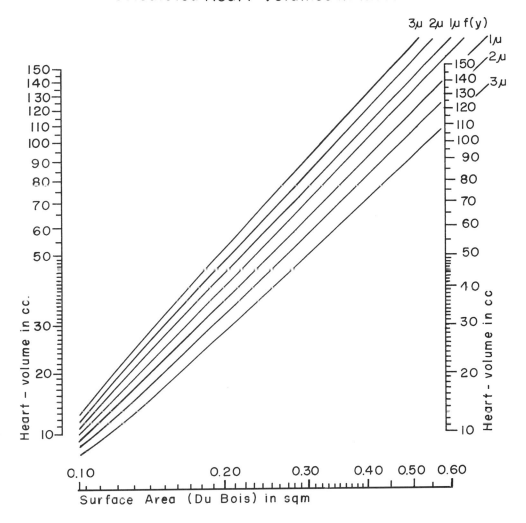

FIG. 182.—(From Lind, J.: Acta radiol., supp. 82, 1950.) *(Continued on next page.)*

MEASUREMENT OF CARDIAC VOLUME

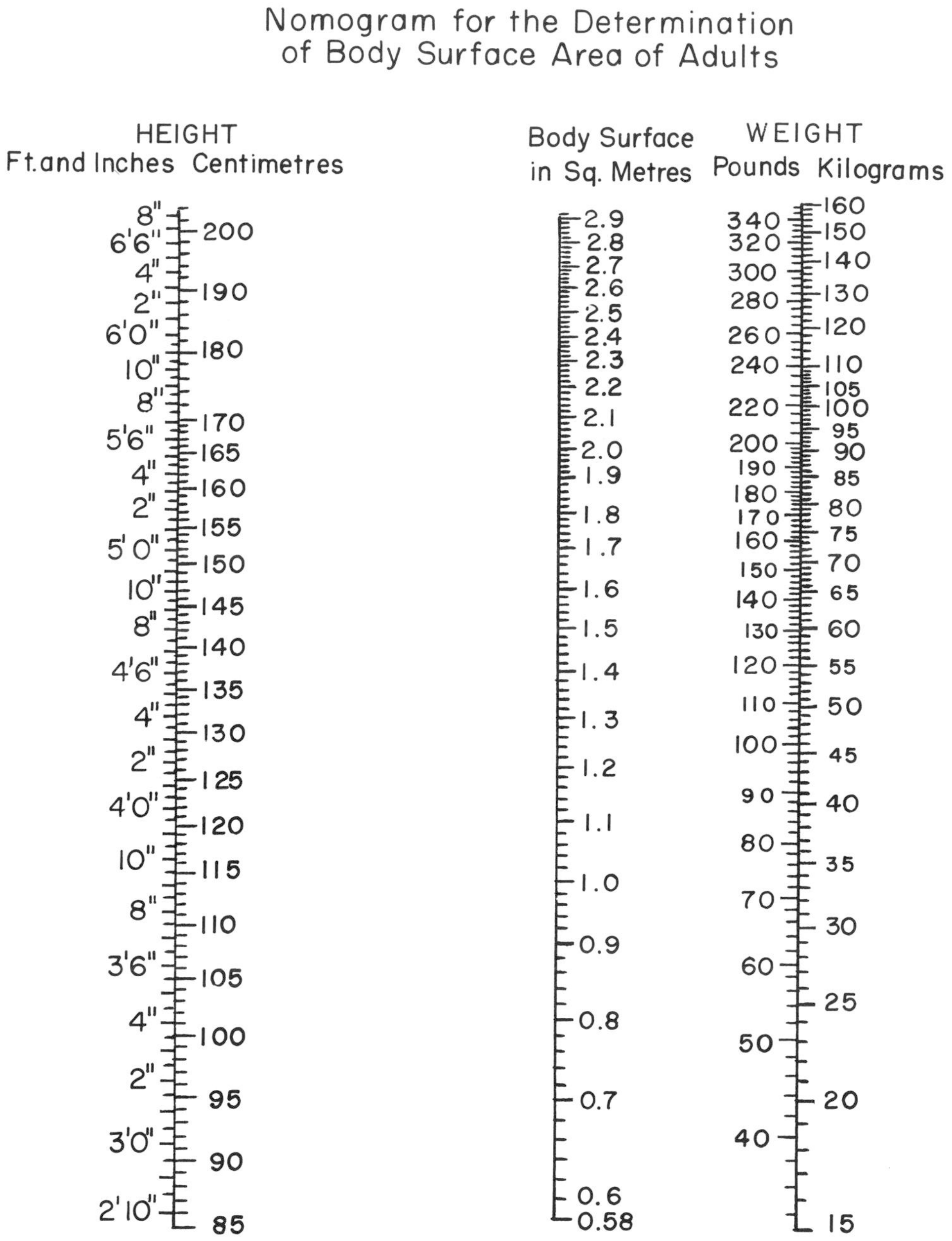
Nomogram for the Determination
of Body Surface Area of Adults
HEIGHT
Ft. and Inches Centimetres
Body Surface
in Sq. Metres
WEIGHT
Pounds Kilograms

FIG. 183.–(Redrawn from Documenta Geigy, *Scientific Tables* [6th ed.; Basel, Switzerland, 1962].)

ADULTS: UPPER LIMITS OF NORMAL*

	Heart Volumes / Body Surface Area =
Females	450–490 cc./m.^{2}
Males	500–540 cc./m.^{2}

*Amundsen, P.: Acta radiol., supp. 181, 1959; Figure 7a.

MEASUREMENT OF CARDIAC VOLUME

1. *Technique*

   a) Central ray: Perpendicular to plane of film centered over midchest.

   b) Position: Posteroanterior in adults and children and anteroposterior or posteroanterior in infants.

   c) Target-film distance: 200 cm. (6 feet), 150 cm. (4 feet 11 inches), or 100 cm. (40 inches).

2. *Measurements*

   See Figures 177 and 178.

   > L = Long diameter. This line extends from the junction of the superior vena cava and right atrium to the cardiac apex.

   > B = Broad diameter. This line extends from the junction of the right atrium and the diaphragm to a point on the left heart border at the junction of the pulmonary artery and left atrial appendage.

   > D = Depth; represents the greatest horizontal depth of the cardiac shadow.

   Calculation of cardiac volume is based on the formula:

   $$V = L \times B \times D \times K$$

   The constant (K) will vary with the focal-film distances used: 200 cm. (6 feet), $K = 0.42$; 150 cm. (4 feet 11 inches), $K = 0.39$; 100 cm. (40 inches), $K = 0.38$.

   The calculated cardiac volume is correlated with body surface area.

   Nomograms for the determination of body surface area for children and adults, derived from patient height and weight, are shown in Figures 181 and 183. The normal heart volumes for infants correlated with body surface area are shown in Figure 182.

   For older children and adults, the variation of normal is sufficiently limited that, for practical purposes, it is adequate to divide the calculated volume by the body surface area and compare with normal standards on page 202.

   Cardiac mensuration by volume determination is probably the most accurate method now available.

3. *Source of Material*

   Nghiem *et al.* studied 305 subjects; 158 were males and 147 were females. Ages ranged from birth to 18 years 9 months. Body surface area ranged from 0.18 to 1.87 m^2 and body weight from 6.2 to 167 lbs.

   Lind's data on normal heart volumes in infants are based on a study of 293 children under 2 years of age, male and female. All were healthy.

   The data on children from 4 to 7, 9 to 12, and 14 to 16 years are taken from Carlgren,* based on a study of 61 healthy children.

   Amundsen's data are based on a study of 87 normal patients — 29 males and 58 females.

---

*Carlgren, L.E.: Acta paediat., vol. 33, supp. 6, 1946.

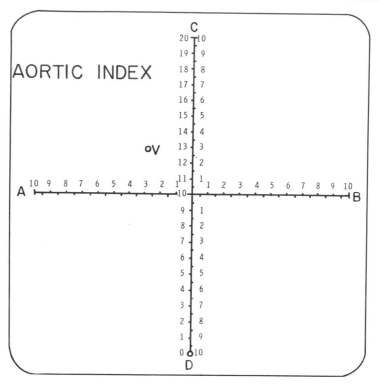

FIG. 184.—Transparent overlay used for determining aortic index. When the overlay is properly centered over the cardiac shadow, *V* is approximately at the aortic valve. (From Lodwick and Gladstone, Fig. 7.)

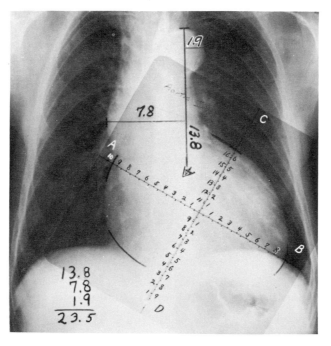

FIG. 185.—Proper centering of overlay on cardiac silhouette. (From Lodwick and Gladstone, Fig. 8.)

*Lodwick, G. S., and Gladstone, W. S.: Radiology 69:70, 1957.

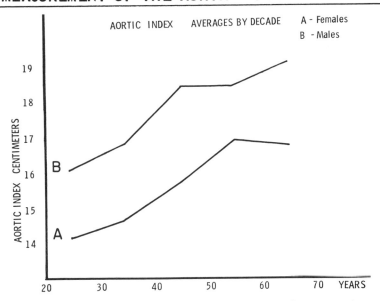

FIG. 186.—Aortic index, averages by decade. *A*, females. *B*, males. (From Lodwick and Gladstone, Fig. 10.)

1. *Technique*

    a) Central ray: Perpendicular to plane of film centered over midportion of chest.

    b) Position: Posteroanterior erect.

    c) Target-film distance: 6 feet.

2. *Measurements*

A transparent overlay is constructed with cross-lines for centering and aligning (Fig. 184). The position of the aortic valve (point *V* on the overlay) bears an approximate relationship to the cross-lines. To measure the aorta, the overlay is placed over the shadow of the cardiac silhouette so that the *AB* axis is aligned with the greatest cardiac dimension. The overlay is adjusted until the numbers on each axis are identical and the cross-lines are at the center of the cardiac silhouette. The hole *V* is now at the estimated site of the aortic valve, and the spot is marked with a wax pencil. The highest and broadest points on the aortic arch are marked on the film, and a vertical reference line is drawn from the highest point downward (Fig. 185). Again using the *AB* and *CD* axes, the height and width of the aortic shadow are determined. These measurements, when totaled, constitute the aortic index.

    Figure 186 gives the aortic index averages by decades. When serologic tests for syphilis are considered in relation to aortic indices in those patients with calcification of the ascending aorta, it is found that 85.1% of all patients with aortic indices greater than 20.0 cm and 100% of all cases with indices in excess of 24.2 cm showed positive serologic evidence of syphilis. It should be noted that in "normal" groups of males, aortic indices do occasionally exceed this figure.

3. *Source of Material*

The "normal" distribution curves for aortic indices of males and females over 20 years of age were constructed from data collected from 228 subjects without clinical evidence of syphilitic aortitis. Sixty-two cases showing calcification in the ascending aorta were also studied by this method.

MEASUREMENT OF LEFT VENTRICULAR CAVITY AND
WALL THICKNESS IN ANGIOCARDIOGRAPHY*

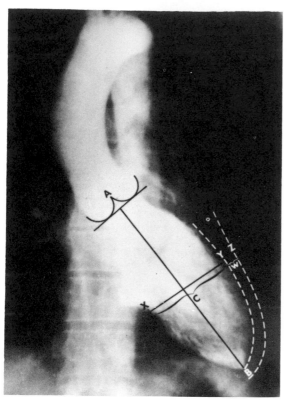

FIG. 187.—(From Levine, Rockoff, and
Braunwald, Fig. 1.)

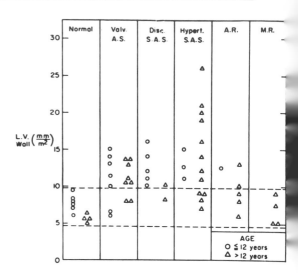

FIG. 188.—(From Levine, Rockoff, and
Braunwald, Fig. 2.)

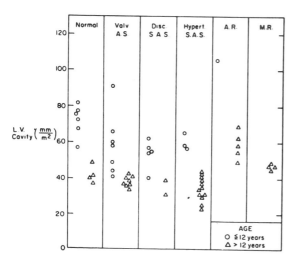

FIG. 189.—(From Levine, Rockoff, and
Braunwald, Fig. 3.)

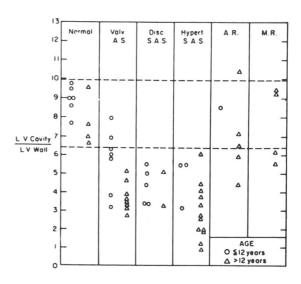

FIG. 190.—(From Levine, Rockoff, and
Braunwald, Fig. 4.)

*Levine, N. D.; Rockoff, D.; and Braunwald, E.: Circulation 28:339, 1963.

MEASUREMENT OF LEFT VENTRICULAR CAVITY AND WALL THICKNESS IN ANGIOCARDIOGRAPHY

1. *Technique*

   a) Central ray: Perpendicular to plane of film centered over midpoint of chest.

   b) Position: Anteroposterior supine.

   c) Target-film distance: 36 inches. Schonander equipment.

2. *Measurements*

   See Figures 187-190.

   Measurements are made on films exposed at the end of diastole.

   AB = Line drawn between the center of the aortic orifice *(A)* and the most distal point of the left ventricular cavity at the apex *(B)*.

   XY = Line drawn perpendicular to AB at its midpoint. The length of XY is taken as the diameter of the left ventricular cavity *(C)*.

   YZ = Lines used to measure the thickness of the free left ventricular wall *(W)*.

   No corrections are made for x-ray distortion, since the error introduced is not felt to be of significance. Results are shown in Figures 188-190. The left ventricular wall thickness in Figures 188 and 189 is corrected for body surface area:

   $$\frac{\text{Measured thickness}}{\text{Body surface area}}$$

   (Normal standards for body surface area are found on pages 200 and 202.)

   In patients with valvular or discrete subvalvular aortic stenosis, the thickness of the free wall of the left ventricle is usually greater than in patients without abnormalities of the left ventricle, and the degree of thickening correlates closely with the degree of obstruction. This type of correlation is not present in patients with hypertrophic subaortic stenosis. No increase in width of the left ventricular cavity is noted in patients with obstruction to left ventricular outflow. In patients with aortic or mitral regurgitations, the width of the left ventricular cavity tended to be increased without any consistent increase in the thickness of the left ventricular wall.

   More detailed methods of analysis of left ventricular chamber volume are found in Dodge, H. T., *et al.*: Am. Heart J. 60:762, 1962; and Figley, M. M.: Radiol. Clin. of North America 2:409, 1964.

3. *Source of Material*

   The data are based on a study of 57 patients, ages 4-52, of whom 35 were age 12 or under. Ten patients had no left ventricular disease; 15 had valvular aortic stenosis; 7 had discrete subvalvular aortic stenosis; 15 had idiopathic hypertrophic subaortic stenosis; 6 had aortic regurgitation; and 4 had mitral regurgitation.

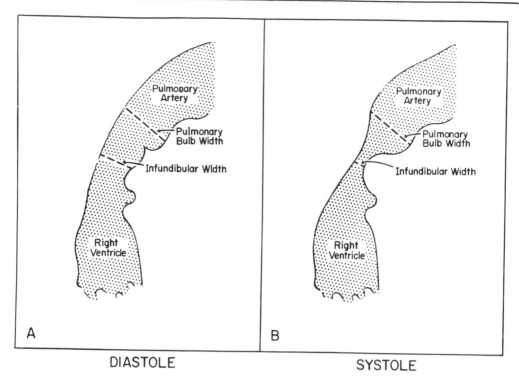

FIG. 191.—(From Little, Fig. 1.*)

A. Infundibular/Bulb Ratio*

Normal range: 0.45-0.83.
        Av. 0.63±0.08.

B. Infundibular Systolic/Diastolic Ratio†

In tetralogy of Fallot: 0:33-1.00.
        Av. 0.56.

In pulmonic valvular stenosis: 0.11-0.30.
        Av. 0.25.

*Little, T. B., *et al.:* Circulation 28:182, 1963.
†Lester, R. G., *et al.:* Am. J. Roentgenol. 94:78, 1965.

MEASUREMENT OF THE INFUNDIBULUM OF THE RIGHT VENTRICLE

1. *Technique*
   a. Central ray: Perpendicular to plane of film centered over midchest.
   b. Projection: True lateral angiocardiograms.
   c. Target-film distance: Immaterial.

2. *Measurements*

   See Figure 191.

   A. The infundibular/bulb ratio. Several bulb measurements are averaged, and the ratio of the minimum systolic diameter to the average pulmonary diameter is obtained. Normal values are given on page 208. The critical ratio is 0.4. Figures below this level indicate significant systolic narrowing.

   B. The infundibular systolic/diastolic ratio. Measurements are made of the infundibulum at its narrowest point in the systole and at the same point in the diastole. In all cases of tetralogy of Fallot, the ratio is greater than 0.33; and in all cases of valvular stenosis, the ratio is less than 0.30. An infundibulum with significant obstruction, as measured by the infundibular/bulb ratio, and an infundibular systolic/diastolic ratio greater than 0.30 may not regress following valvulotomy.

3. *Source of Material*

   The data on the infundibular/bulb ratio are based on a study of 13 patients with pulmonary valvular stenosis and 30 control subjects.

   The infundibular systolic diameter/infundibular diastolic ratio is based on a study of 42 patients with tetralogy of Fallot and 19 patients with pulmonic valvular stenosis.

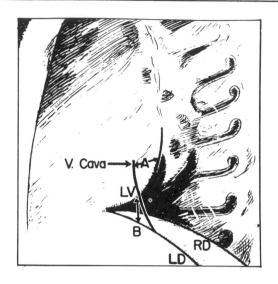

FIG. 192.–(From Hoffman, R. B., and Rigler, L. G.:
Radiology 85:93, 1965, Fig. 2.)

LV = left ventricle
V. Cava = inferior vena cava
RD = right diaphragm
LD = left diaphragm

VENA CAVAL–LEFT VENTRICULAR RELATIONSHIPS IN HEART DISEASE

1. Technique

   a) Central ray: Perpendicular to plane of film centered over midchest.

   b) Position: True lateral. Full inspiration.

   c) Target-film distance: 6 feet.

2. Measurements

See Figure 192.

    With full inspiration and in true lateral projection, the shadow of the interior vena cava in the retrocardiac space is not completely included in the cardiac silhouette. Eyler and his associates* have shown that this relationship is useful in differentiating mitral stenosis from mitral insufficiency. With mitral insufficiency, the left ventricle projects behind the shadow of the inferior vena cava for a distance of 15 mm. or more.

    Keats and Rudhe[†] use this relationship in differentiating atrial secundum septal defect from ventricular septal defects. In the atrial secundum septal defect, the inferior vena cava lies in part free in the retrocardiac space. In the ventricular septal defect, with large shunt, the vena cava is projected over the mass of the heart.

    Hoffman and Rigler[‡] have defined two additional measurements for determining left ventricular enlargement. Measurement A, Figure 192, is defined as the distance which the left ventricle *(LV)* extends posteriorly to the posterior border of the inferior vena cava (v. cava) at a point 2 cm. cephalad to the crossing of the cava and the left ventricle. This measurement is made on a plane extending posteriorly which parallels the horizontal plan of the vertebral bodies. Measurement B is the distance of this crossing caudad to the left leaf of the diaphragm. When A is more than 1.8 cm., one can postulate left ventricular enlargement with a considerable degree of certainty. When B is less than 0.75 cm., one can suspect left ventricular enlargement.

3. Source of Material

    Eyler's data are based on a study of 214 cases of rheumatic heart disease, surgically explored.

    Keats and Rudhe's data are based on a study of 32 patients with atrial secundum defects, ages 9-28 years; 36 patients with ventricular septal defects, ages 4-32 years; and 30 normal subjects, ages 4-36 years.

    Hoffman and Rigler's data are based on a study of 270 subjects, including 122 normals, the remainder being patients with aortic and mitral valvular diseases and hypertension.

---

*Eyler, W. R., *et al.:* Radiology 73:56, 1959.
[†]Keats, T. E., and Rudhe, U.: Radiology 83:616, 1964.
[‡]Hoffman, R. B., and Rigler, L. G.: Radiology 85:93, 1965.

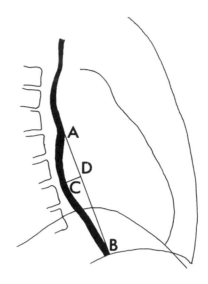

FIG. 193.—(Redrawn from Kaye *et al.*, Fig. 4.)

1. Technique

a) Central ray: Perpendicular to plane of film centered over midpoint of chest.

b) Position: Right anterior oblique with barium outlining the esophagus. Optimum degree of rotation determined during fluoroscopy. Full inspiration.

c) Target-film distance: 64 inches.

2. Measurements

See Figure 193.

Line *AB* is drawn from the anterior aspect of the esophagus where it begins a backward sweep at the upper level of the left atrium to a point on the anterior aspect of the esophagus where it passes the left leaf on the diaphragm, or any more anterior portion above this point.

Line *CD* is the posterior displacement of the esophagus. Line *CD* is drawn perpendicular to Line *AB* at the maximum displacement of the esophagus. The distance *CD* is measured in millimeters from Line *AB* to the anterior wall of the esophagus.

POSTERIOR DISPLACEMENT OF THE ESOPHAGUS IN THE ERECT ANTERIOR OBLIQUE VIEW

	Mean Displacement	Standard Deviation	± 2 Standard Deviations
Normal	7.9 mm.	3.0 mm.	2-14 mm.
Mitral value disease	19.6 mm.	10.4 mm.	0-40 mm.

3. Source of Material

Fifty normal subjects and 50 patients with mitral valve disease. The diagnosis was based on clinical electrocardiographic and phonocardiographic findings. Age and sex incidence were similar in both groups.

---

*Kaye, J., *et al.*: Brit. J. Radiol. 28:693, 1955.

A. In Children

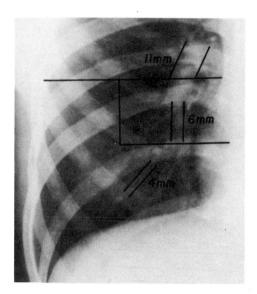

FIG. 194.—(From Leinbach, Fig. 1.)

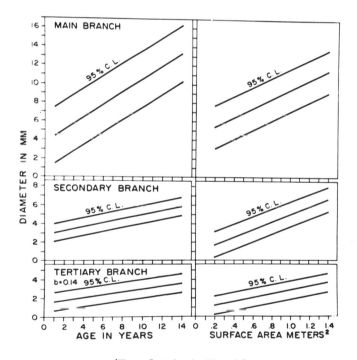

(From Leinbach, Fig. 2.)

*Leinbach, L. B.: Am. J. Roentgenol. 89:995, 1963.

MEASUREMENT OF THE NORMAL PULMONARY ARTERIES

A. In Children

1. *Technique*

   a) Central ray: Perpendicular to plane of film centered over midchest.

   b) Position: Posteroanterior.

   c) Target-film distance: 6 feet.

2. *Measurements*

   See Figure 194.

   The right lower lung field is utilized. A horizontal line is drawn from the descending branch of the right pulmonary artery just below the right hilar shadow to the lateral chest wall. A perpendicular line is then drawn inferiorly from the midpoint of this line to meet a horizontal line drawn bisecting the distance from the upper line and the cardiophrenic reflection. In this way, a central square-shaped area and a peripheral L-shaped area are obtained. Three measurements are made: (1) the diameter of the right descending pulmonary artery is measured as it appears below the right hilus; (2) the diameter of the widest-caliber secondary arterial branch is measured in the central area; and (3) the widest tertiary branch is then measured in the peripheral area. Normal measurements on function of age and surface area are shown in the chart below Figure 194. Normal values for surface area are found on page 200.

3. *Source of Material*

   The data are based on a study of 243 children ranging in age from infancy to 14 years. Each chest film used was interpreted as normal with the diaphragmatic level at least the 9th posterior rib.

B. In Adults

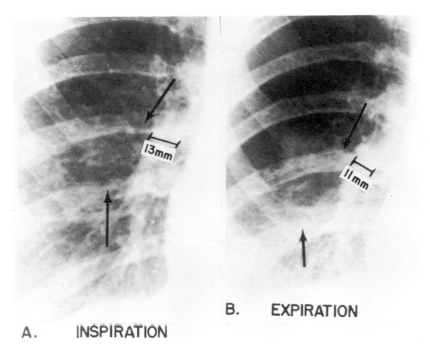

FIG. 195.—(From Chang, C. H.: Am. J. Roentgenol. 87:929, 1962.)

	INSPIRATION	EXPIRATION	RANGE OF DIFFERENCE BETWEEN INSPIRATION AND EXPIRATION
Males	16 mm.	15 mm.	1-3 mm.
Females	15 mm.	14 mm.	1-3 mm.

(From Chang.)

B. In Adults

1. *Technique*

  a) Central ray: Perpendicular to plane of film centered over midchest.
  b) Position: Posteroanterior.
  c) Target-film distance: 6 feet.

2. *Measurements*

See Figure 195.

All films are obtained in deep inspiration and forceful expiration. The right descending pulmonary artery is measured on both inspiratory and expiratory films at its widest point near the bifurcation of the artery from the lateral segment of the right middle lobe and above the branching of the middle basilar artery. This measurement point usually lies between the right 8th and 9th ribs posteriorly in deep inspirations. On expiration, it usually lies just below or over the right 8th rib posteriorly.

Normal values are shown in the chart. Values greater than those shown are abnormal, and pulmonary hypertension is most likely present.* The expiratory measurement is always smaller than the inspiratory, and it is helpful in borderline cases.

These measurements are also useful in the diagnosis of pulmonary infarction.[†] With infarction, values ranging from 17 to 22 mm. are noted on the right, and from 17 to 26 mm. on the left, on inspiration. This dilatation usually appears within 24 hours of the onset of chest pain, and maximum dilatation occurs in 2-3 days.

3. *Source of Material*

The data on normal size are based on a study of 1,085 normal adults, including 432 males ranging in age from 18 to 70 years and 652 females ranging from 18 to 72 years.

Figures for pulmonary infarction are based on a study of 23 patients with pulmonary infarction.

---

*Chang, C. H.: Am. J. Roentgenol. 87:929, 1962.
[†]Chang, C. H., and Davis, W. C.: Clin. Radiol. 16:141, 1965.

MEASUREMENT OF THE SIZE OF THE ARCH OF THE AZYGOUS VEIN*

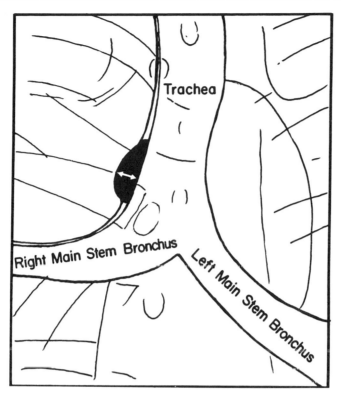

FIG. 196.—(From Keats and Lipscomb.)

NORMAL VALUES

Minimum	3 mm.
Maximum	7 mm.
Average	4.9 mm.

1. *Technique*

   a) Central ray: Perpendicular to plane of film centered over midchest.
   b) Position: Posteroanterior, upright; inspiratory phase of respiration.
   c) Target-film distance: 72 inches.

2. *Measurements*

   See Figure 196.

   The width of the azygous arches is measured perpendicularly to the trachea in the greatest transverse dimension of the arch. Measurement includes the wall of the trachea.

   The normal ranges are exceeded in pregnancy, congestive heart failure, portal hypertension, and obstructions of the superior or inferior vena cava.

3. *Source of Material*

   The data are based on a study of 200 normal adults, equally divided between males and females between the ages of 20 and 60 years.

*Keats, T. E., and Lipscomb, G.: Radiology 90:990, 1968.

WIDTH OF THE AZYGOS VEIN RELATED TO
CENTRAL VENOUS PRESSURE*

1. *Technique*

   a) Central ray: Perpendicular to plane of film centered over midchest.
   b) Position: Anteroposterior. Patient supine on bed rolled flat. Maximum inspiration phase of respiration.
   c) Target-film distance: 40 inches.

2. *Measurements*

   See Figure 196.
   The azygos vein width is measured at its greatest diameter, perpendicular to the wall of the trachea. This measurement includes the mediastinal pleural reflection laterally and the tracheal wall medially.

Width of Azygos Vein (mm.)	Estimated CVP (to nearest cm.)	95% Confidence Limits (to nearest cm.)
4	3	0-10
6	5	0-12
8	8	1-15
10	11	4-18
12	14	7-21
14	17	10-24
16	19	12-26
18	22	15-29
20	25	18-32
22	28	21-35
24	31	24-38
26	33	26-40
28	36	29-43

(From Preger *et al.*, Table 1.)

3. *Source of Material*

   Fifty-four adult patients ranging in age from 23 to 77 years of age. In this group were patients with congestive heart failure, patients recovering from thoracic surgery and recipients of renal transplants.

---

*Preger, L., *et al.:* Radiology 93:521, 1969.

ANATOMIC LEVEL OF ORIGIN OF AORTIC BRANCHES*

RELATIONSHIP BETWEEN VERTEBRAL BODIES AND ORIGIN OF AORTIC BRANCHES
(After Caldwell)†

ARTERY	RANGE	MEAN	RANGE FOR 85% OF PATIENTS
Celiac	UT11 to UL2	UL1	MT12 to DL1-2
Superior mesenteric	MT12 to DL2-3	LL1	UL1 to UL2
Right renal	LT12 to ML4	UL2	LL1 to ML2
Left renal	MT12 to ML4	UL2	LL1 to ML2
Inferior mesenteric	ML2 to LL4	LL3	UL3 to UL4
Aortic bifurcation	ML3 to LL5	LL4	UL4 to UL5

†Symbols: U, upper; M, middle; and L, lower portions of the thoracic (T) and lumbar (L) vertebrae. Discs (D) are designated in reference to the vertebral bodies they separate.

Source of Material

The data are based on dissections of 300 consecutive cadavers of American Caucasians and Negroes, ranging in age from 18 to 78 years. Twenty-three were females. The data are useful for catheter positioning in selective and nonselective abdominal aortography.

*Seitchik, M. W., et al.: Surg., Gynec., & Obst. 160:192, 1960.

†Caldwell, E. W., and Anson, B. J.: Am. J. Anat. 73:27, 1943.

MEASUREMENT OF THE ABDOMINAL AORTA*

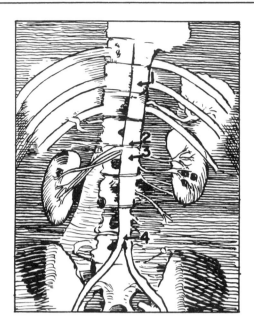

FIG. 197.—(From Steinberg, Fig. 1.)

AVERAGE AGE AND DIAMETER IN MM. OF ABDOMINAL AORTA AT SITES MEASURED*

Sex and Diagnosis	No. of Cases	Age	At 11th Rib	Above Renal Arteries	Below Renal Arteries	At Bifurcation of Aorta	Difference between 11th Rib and Bifurcation of Aorta
Male							
Normal	29	53.9±13.7	26.9±3.96	23.9±3.92	21.4± 3.65	18.7± 3.34	8.14± 2.14
Hypertensive	49	48.6±15.1	27.7±4.62	24.5±4.43	21.3± 4.37	19.5± 3.08	8.16± 3.70
Occlusive	109	56.8± 9.9	27.2±3.42	23.6±3.29	20.5± 3.30	18.2± 3.68	9.08± 3.72
Abdominal aneurysm	90	63.6± 7.1	33.5±6.05	31.2±8.36	34.3±12.56	31.8±10.53	1.76±10.23
Female							
Normal	44	56.9±14.3	24.4±3.45	21.6±3.16	18.7± 3.36	17.5± 2.52	6.80± 4.54
Hypertensive	45	53.8±13.0	25.6±2.85	21.7±3.02	19.5± 3.29	17.5± 2.92	8.09± 2.22
Occlusive	48	57.0± 8.5	24.7±2.96	20.7±2.71	17.6± 2.74	15.7± 3.02	8.92± 3.48
Abdominal aneurysm	18	67.2± 7.3	30.5±6.05	28.5±6.94	32.2±14.00	25.4± 6.21	5.05± 6.40

(From Steinberg, Table I.)

*Steinberg, C. R., *et al.:* Am. J. Roentgenol. 95:703, 1965.

MEASUREMENT OF THE ABDOMINAL AORTA

1. *Technique*

   a) Central ray: Perpendicular to plane of film centered over midabdomen.
   b) Position: Anteroposterior.
   c) Target-film distance: 48 inches.

2. *Measurements*

   See Figure 197.

   Measurements were made at the following sites:

   1. The 11th rib, the level where the aorta pierces the diaphragm.
   2. Above the renal arteries, at a site which is almost at one half the length of the abdominal aorta and is below the celiac axis.
   3. Below the renal arteries.
   4. At the bifurcation of the abdominal aorta.

   The values for male and female normals, hypertensives, and patients with occlusive arterial disease and abdominal aneurysms are given in the table below Figure 197. Hypertension and thrombotic occlusive disease do not alter the mean diameter. In arteriosclerotic aneurysmal disease, there is enlargement of the aorta at each site, suggesting that aortic dilatation is a significant accompaniment of the aneurysm.

3. *Source of Material*

   Measurements are based on a study of 500 consecutive patients referred for intravenous abdominal aortography.

VI. THE GASTROINTESTINAL SYSTEM

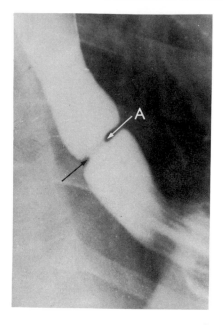

FIG. 198.—(From Schatzki, Fig. 2A.†)

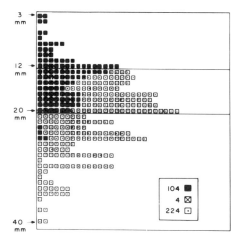

■ Dysphagia,
  repeated episodes

⊠ Dysphagia,
  single episode

☐ No dysphagia

104	■
4	⊠
224	☐

Chart showing relationship between dysphagia and diameter of esophageal rings of various patients. The measurement refers to the maximal diameter of the ring at the time of first demonstration as measured on spot roentgenogram. (From Schatzki, Fig. 1.†)

*Schatzki, R., and Gary, J. W.: Am. J. Roentgenol. 70:911, 1953.

†Schatzki, R.: Am. J. Roentgenol. 90: 805, 1963.

MEASUREMENT OF THE LOWER ESOPHAGEAL RING

1. *Technique*

   a) Central ray: Spot roentgenograms are used.

   b) Position: Erect or recumbent.

   c) Target-film distance: Variable. Target-table top distance: 18 inches.

2. *Measurements*

   See Figure 198.

   Maximum diameter of the ring in a barium-filled esophagus. Measured on spot films without consideration of magnification.

   Schatzki states that the lower esophageal ring:

   a) Is not a abnormal contraction.

   b) Lies at the junction of esophageal and gastric mucosa and is the junction of esophagus and stomach.

   c) Which has an original diameter of less than 13 mm. has always been symptomatic in his experience.

3. *Source of Material*

   The data are based on measurements of 104 patients with repeated episodes of dysphagia, 4 patients with one episode of dysphagia, and 224 patients without dysphagia. *Note:* This does not include all asymptomatic patients with lower esophageal ring who were seen in this study.

MEASUREMENT OF ESOPHAGEAL DIAMETER*

MEASUREMENT MADE AT THE LEVEL OF THE
CRICOPHARYNGEUS MUSCLE

AGE	ANATOMIC DIAM. (Mm.)
9 days to 4 weeks	6
1-9 months	7-8
10 months to 7 years	8-11
7-16 years	9-13

1. *Technique*

   a) Central ray: Spot roentgenograms are used.

   b) Position: Lateral neck. Erect or recumbent position. Barium-filled esophagus.

   c) Target-film distance: Variable. Roentgenographic measurements must be corrected before comparison is made with above table.

2. *Measurements*

   The cricopharyngeal diameter was found to be the narrowest point. Range of measurements is shown in above table.

3. *Source of Material*

   Fresh esophageal specimens were obtained from 28 cadavers. Direct measurement of mucosa was made. In no case was the cause of death due to an abnormality of the esophagus.

---

*Haase, F. R., and Brenner, A.: Arch. Otolaryng. 77:119, 1963.

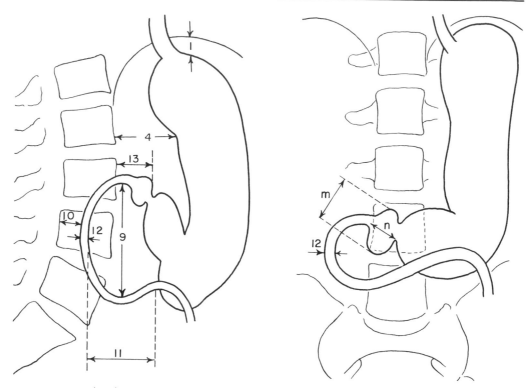

FIG. 199 (left).—Stomach and duodenum in right lateral recumbent or left lateral erect positions. (Redrawn from Meschan *et al.*)

FIG. 200 (right).—Stomach and duodenum in posteroanterior recumbent position. (Redrawn from Meschan *et al.*)

1. Technique

   a) Central ray: Posteroanterior recumbent—To 2d lumbar vertebra.

   Right lateral recumbent—3 inches anterior to midcoronal plane at level of 2d lumbar vertebra.

   Left lateral erect—Same as right lateral recumbent. Stomach may be lower in position than for recumbent, and fluoroscopic observation is recommended for accurate centering.

   b) Position: Posteroanterior recumbent.

   Right lateral recumbent.

   Left lateral erect.

   c) Target-film distance: 36 inches.

   Stomach contained approximately 8 ounces of barium sulfate in water. Films obtained in suspended respiration.

2. Measurements

   See Figures 199 and 200.

   1 = Distance between top of stomach fundus and diaphragm.

   4 = Stomach to anterior spine. See measurements on retrogastric space, page 229.

   9 = Maximum vertical internal diameter of the duodenal loop.

   10 = Minimum measurement of the outer margin of the second portion of the duodenum to the posterior margin of the vertebral bodies.

*Meschan, I., *et al.*: South. M. J. 46:878, 1953.

RELATIONSHIPS OF STOMACH AND DUODENUM TO THE
SPINE IN DIFFERENT WEIGHT AND STOMACH TYPE GROUPS
(BOTH ASYMPTOMATIC AND SYMPTOMATIC SUMMATED)

Weight Group	Stomach Type	No. of Cases	9 Rt. Lat. Avg. of Medians	9 Rt. Lat. Range	10 Rt. Lat. Avg. of Medians	10 Rt. Lat. Range	11 Rt. Lat. Avg. of Medians	11 Rt. Lat. Range	13 Rt. Lat. Avg. of Medians	13 Rt. Lat. Range
NORMAL	J-shape	58	6.5	4.0-9.5	3.0	1.0-9.0	3.0	0.0-12.5	4.0	0.5-8.0
	Fish-hook	10	6.0	4.0-8.0	3.0	2.5-4.0	5.6	3.5-8.0	4.5	2.5-9.0
	Cascade	13	6.0	4.5-6.0	4.3	2.0-9.5	6.6	1.0-11.0	6.0	2.5-9.0
	Steer-horn	9	6.5	5.5-8.0	3.5	0.5-5.0	5.5	1.5-9.0	5.0	2.5-10.0
UNDER WT	J-shape	56	5.5	2.0-11.0	3.0	0.5-7.0	4.0	0.0-9.0	3.0	0.5-6.5
	Fish-hook	21	5.5	3.5-8.0	2.5	0.0-5.0	3.0	1.5-5.0	2.5	1.0-4.0
	Cascade	5	6.0	5.5-6.5	2.5	2.0-3.5	4.5	4.0-5.0	3.0	2.0-5.0
	Steer-horn	3	8.0	8.0	4.5	2.0-6.0	7.0	6.5-8.0	4.0	1.5-5.0
OVER WT	J-shape	13	6.5	4.0-9.0	3.3	2.0-7.0	4.5	3.5-9.0	3.5	1.5-9.5
	Fish-hook	5	5.0	3.0-7.5	2.5	0.0-4.0	4.5	2.0-9.5	4.6	3.0-6.5
	Cascade	10	7.0	4.0-9.0	4.0	1.0-7.5	5.0	1.5-10.0	5.6	3.0-12.0
	Steer-horn	8	6.0	5.5-8.0	4.0	3.5-5.5	5.0	3.0-7.5	4.5	3.0-7.5

211

(Data from Meschan *et al.*)

11 = Maximum horizontal internal diameter of the duodenal loop.
12 = Maximum outer diameter of the second portion of the duodenum.
13 = Distance between pylorus and the outer margin of the spine.
m = Width of base of duodenal bulb.
n = Height of duodenal bulb from apex to pylorus.

Figure 199, dimension *l:* Av. = 0.5 cm.; max. = 1.5 cm.
Diameter of second portion of duodenum, Figures 199 and 200, dimension *12:*

Av. = 2.0 cm.; min. = 1.0 cm.; max. = 2.5 cm.
Width of gastric and duodenal rugae:
Upper stomach, 0.5 cm.
Lower stomach, 0.3-0.5 cm.
Midduodenum, 0.2-0.3 cm.
Size of duodenal bulb (Fig. 200):
    m = Width at base   Av. = 3.0 cm.; max. = 3.5 cm.
    n = Height   Av. = 3.0 cm.; max. = 4.0 cm.

Types of stomachs:

J-shaped or eutonic stomach: Pylorus and incisura angularis are at the same level.

Cascade stomach: Fundus has a posterior pouchlike projection which overlaps the body of the stomach.

Fishhook or hypotonic type stomach: Incisura angularis is considerably lower than pylorus.

Steer-horn stomach: Incisura angularis lies above the level of the pylorus.

Weight Groups:

See table on page 227.

Meschan *et al.* divided the patients into three groups according to weight. The Equitable Life Assurance Society standards for height and weight were used to establish whether patients were normal weight (plus or minus 10%), overweight, or underweight.

3. *Source of Material*

The data are based on a study of 211 adult individuals of all ages between the third and the seventh decade, chosen at random from two Veterans Administration Hospitals, University of Arkansas Hospital, and University of Arkansas medical students.

Of these adults, 107 were asymptomatic and 104 were symptomatic with no apparent radiographic abnormality in stomach or duodenum.

Sex and age distribution were random.

Over 10,000 measurements were made for this study.

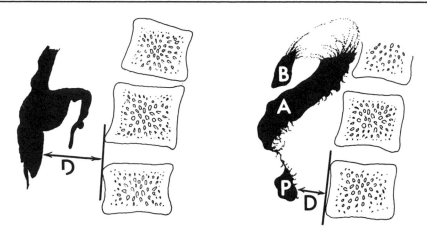

FIG. 201.　　　　　　　　　　　　FIG. 202.

(Redrawn from Poole, Figs. 4 and 5.)

1. Technique

a) Central ray: To barium-filled stomach and duodenum during fluoroscopic examination.

b) Position: Left lateral erect. Patient's left shoulder toward fluoroscopic screen, right shoulder against table top.

c) Target-film distance: Varies with thickness of patient. A coin marker, for instance a nickel, is placed on the skin for purposes of magnification correction.

2. Measurements

See Figures 201 and 202.

A barium mixture of 3 parts Intropaque, 2 parts Barosperse, and 5 parts water (all by volume) were used by Poole. In the upright posteroanterior position the patient swallows ½ oz. of barium.

Antrum-to-Spine Measurement. See Figure 201. The fluoroscopic pressure cone is used to flatten the column of barium in the antrum. Adequate compression is denoted by displacement of the barium column to both sides of the midline.

The patient is then turned laterally with arms raised so that his right side is against the table top and the spot-film device is against his left side. A compression device (Poole used a plunger-type device with a padded head 3½ inches in diameter) is placed over the same spot on the anterior abdominal wall as was used in splaying the folds in the posteroanterior projection. The patient is fluoroscoped and the abdominal wall is pressed with the compression device until the midline viscus strikes the retroperitoneal structures. A lateral spot-film is taken. Distance D is measured as shown in Figure 201 from the posterior stomach wall to the anterior vertebral body surface. Distance is corrected for magnification according to the following ratio:

$$\frac{D_t}{D_m} = \frac{C_t}{C_m}; \ D_t = \frac{D_m C_t}{C_m}$$

---

*Poole, G. J.: Radiology 97:71, 1970.

where:

D_t = True antrum- or duodenum-to-spine distance;
D_m = Magnified distance from antrum or duodenum to spine measured on the spot-film;
C_t = True marker diameter (nickel coin);
C_m = Magnified marker's greatest diameter measured on the spot-film.

Corrected antrum-to-spine distance is plotted against weight as shown below in Figure 203.

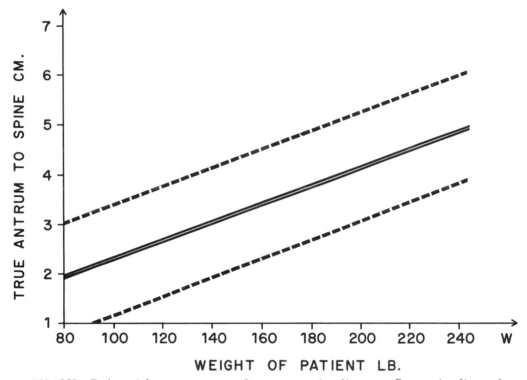

FIG. 203.—Body weight versus corrected antrum-to-spine distance. Regression line and 95% confidence limits are shown. (From Poole, Fig. 9.)

Duodenum-to-Spine Measurement. See Figure 202. Following the antrum-to-spine spot-film, the patient is placed in the right lateral decubitus position to allow barium to enter the horizontal duodenum. The patient is placed erect in the posteroanterior position. When the midline duodenum is identified the patient is turned to a left lateral position. When the horizontal duodenum is seen on end, a spot-film is made without pressure. The duodenum-to-spine distance is measured from the posterior aspect of the midline duodenum to the spine (measurement D, Fig. 202). If hypertrophic spurs are present, the measurement is taken to the anterior aspect of the spurs. Measurement D is corrected for magnification as described for antrum-to-spine measurement.

Mean value is 1.3 cm. (S.D. 5 mm.)
Upper limit of normal is 2.3 cm. (1.3 cm. + 2 S.D.).
The duodenum-to-spine measurement showed no relationship to body weight.

3. *Source of Material*

Antrum-to-spine measurements were made on 141 patients who had no radiographic or clinical evidence of retrogastric mass. Duodenum-to-spine measurements were made on 96 patients who had no radiographic or clinical evidence of retrogastric mass.

PROBABILITY TABLES FOR RADIOLOGIC DIAGNOSIS

What future developments in quantitative radiology might be expected to follow data collection from static images? Several suggestions have been made recently.* We would like to propose that a useful next step would be collection and analysis of roentgen data to construct "public models" as an aid to roentgen diagnosis. A public model (statistical or otherwise) is one that commands general agreement among scientists about a situation in which data are obtained. A specific type of public model for roentgen diagnosis, based on the data of W. J. Wilson, is shown on the following page. The purpose of the public model is to try to reduce disagreement and uncertainty among radiologists about the definition, appearance and probability of radiologic observations. The material is presented in the form of sample probability tables to aid the radiologist with diagnosis.

On the left side of the page the definition of a sign is given and a drawing or a picture is presented, if appropriate. If disagreement about a definition or drawing exists among radiologists it is easier to focus on the disagreement by using this method. Conversely, specific definitions and illustrations should make final agreement among radiologists easier to reach. On the right side of the page probabilities are presented which represent the experience of one group of investigators. The radiologist can use the likelihood ratios as weighting factors which added together give an indication of the benign or malignant state of the ulcer.

As more public models and probability tables are developed they could be compiled in handbook form for the radiologist. We would appreciate the comments and suggestions of readers concerning public models and probability tables. Our publisher, Year Book Medical Publishers, Inc., was generous enough to allow insertion of this page and the public model page on an experimental basis in the *Atlas*

---

*Symposium on Quantitative Data Derived from Radiologic Images. Saratoga Springs, N.Y., May 1971, Invest. Radiol. July-Aug. 1972.

GASTRIC ULCER—BENIGN VS. MALIGNANT

Diagnosis (Prior Probability or Incidence)	Benign 0.75	Malignant 0.25	Likelihood Ratio
Sign or Symptom	Probability $P(S/D_1)$	Probability $P(S/D_2)$	$= \dfrac{P(S/D_2)}{P(S/D_1)}$
1. Adjacent mass	0.01	0.42	42.0
2. Ulcer shape asymmetric	0.01	0.33	33.0
3. Rugal folds absent	0.01	0.24	24.0
4. Crater margin nodular	0.04	0.60	15.0
5. Gastric wall rigidity	0.10	0.80	8.0
6. Ulcer crater base 6 mm. or more inside gastric wall	0.13	0.74	6.0

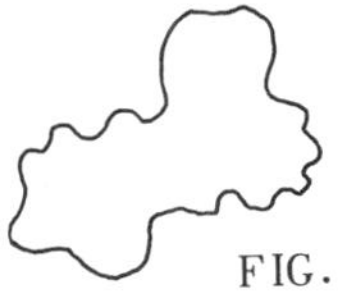

FIG. 204.

FIG. 205.

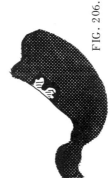

FIG. 206.

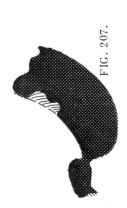

FIG. 207.

Definition of Sign

1. Adjacent mass is a nodular, an irregular, or an asymmetric filling defect associated with the crater. The presence of a mass excludes a mound.

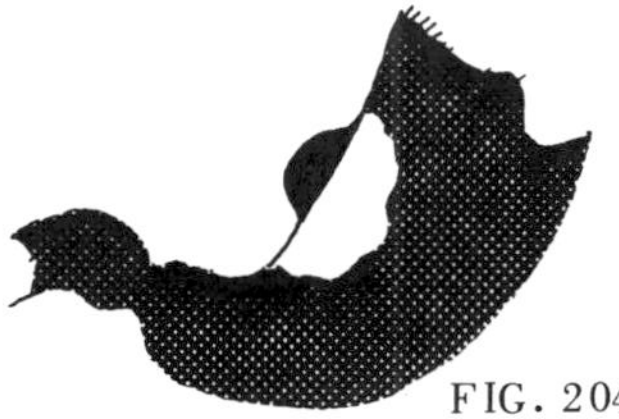

2. Ulcer shape asymmetric.

4. Crater margin nodular.

6. Crater base 6 mm. or more inside gastric wall.

*Wilson, W. J., *et al.:* Radiology 85:1064, 1965.

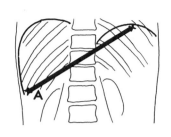

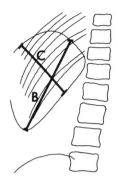

FIG. 208.   FIG. 209.

(Redrawn from Walk,* Figs. 2 and 3.)

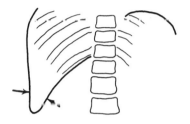

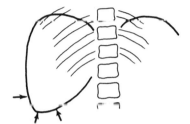

FIG. 210.—Thin border of liver.   FIG. 211.—Rounded border of liver.

(Redrawn from Walk,* Figs. 5 and 6.)

1. Technique

a) Central ray: Centered over upper abdomen.

b) Position: Exposure 1 is taken anteroposterior with patient supine. (Figure 208.)
   Exposure 2 is taken in right posterior oblique position of 50° to 60°.
   (Fig. 209.)

c) Target-film distance: 120 cm.

2. Measurements

See Figures 208 and 209.

Dimension A (Fig. 208) is the distance from the right border of the liver to the middle of the left cupola of the diaphragm. Use Exposure 1.

Dimension B (Fig. 209) is the distance from the antero=inferior border of the liver to the most distal part of its posterior surface as outlined by the diaphragm. Use Exposure 2.

Dimension C (Fig. 209) is the distance from the posterior surface of the liver, where it lies close to the upper pole of the kidney, to the upper anterior surface. Use Exposure 2.

*Walk, L.: Acta radiol. 55:49, 1961.
†Walk, L.: Acta radiol. (Diagnosis) 6:369, 1967.

DETERMINATION OF LIVER VOLUME*†

For a target-film distance of 120 cm. the A, B and C dimensions taken from the two exposures are used in the following formula:

$$\text{Liver volume} = A \cdot B \cdot C \text{ index}$$

Indices to be used for children and adults are shown below for normal border, thin border (see Fig. 210), and round border (see Fig. 211).

INDICES TO BE USED FOR CHILDREN IN CALCULATION OF LIVER VOLUME.*

Age of patient	Liver configuration		
	Round border	Normal border	Thin border
1 year	0.242	0.217	0.204
2-3 yrs	0.227	0.204	0.191
4-6 yrs	0.215	0.193	0.181
7-11 yrs	0.204	0.183	0.172
12-17 yrs	0.197	0.177	0.166

INDICES TO BE USED FOR ADULTS IN CALCULATION OF LIVER VOLUME.

Rounded border	0.19
Normal configuration	0.17
Thin border	0.16

Liver volume per square meter of body surface is clinically useful. Surface area is calculated according to the formula of DuBois and DuBois,† as follows:

$$\text{Body surface area } (m^2) = \text{Weight} \frac{1}{2.35} (\text{kg.}) \times \text{Height} \frac{1}{1.38} (\text{cm.}) \times 6$$

Normal liver volume = 850 cc./m².
Borderline liver volume = 800-900 cc./m².
Liver volume over 900 cc./m² is definitely pathologic.

3. Source of Material

Roentgenologic measurements of the liver were compared with the postmortem specimen measurements in 80 autopsies. Error was ±16%.

*Walk, L.: Acta radiol. (Diagnosis) 6:369, 1967.

†DuBois, D., and DuBois, E. F.: Proc. Soc. Exper. Biol. & Med. 13:77, 1916.

MEASUREMENT OF THE WIDTHS OF THE PORTAL AND SPLENIC VEIN*

1. Technique

    a) Central ray: Centered over spleen.

    b) Position: Anteroposterior abdomen.

    c) Target-film distance: 100 cm.

    Films taken in deep inspiration.

    Thirty cc. of Triurol 50% (sodium acetrizoate: specific gravity, 1.3; viscosity at 37° C., 2.1 centipoise) was injected into the spleen at the rate of 6-7.5 cc./sec. Films were taken with an automatic film changer at a rate of 1 film per second for 13 seconds after the beginning of the injection; then 1 film every 3 seconds for 20 seconds.

2. Measurements

    Diameter of the splenic vein (measured hepatoproximally, where the vein usually is of uniform width) = less than 16 mm.

    Diameter of the portal vein (measured hepatodistally, where the vein is widest = less than 23 mm.

    Note: No correction was made for variation in vessel-film distance with body build.

3. Source of Material

    The data are based on a study of 14 adults with no evidence of portal hypertension. The widths of the splenic vein and the portal vein are often increased in the presence of portal hypertension.

---

*Bergstrand, I., and Eckman, C.-A.: Acta radiol. 47:1, 1957.

MEASUREMENT OF COMMON BILE DUCT DIAMETER

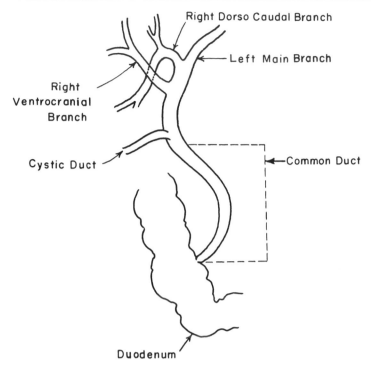

FIG. 212.

1. *Technique*

   a) Central ray: To 12th thoracic vertebra on median plane.

   b) Position: Posteroanterior, rolled up 15° toward the right; additional
   projections obtained as necessary after inspecting scout
   film.

   Posteroanterior tomograms may be necessary.

   First tomogram is taken by setting the fulcrum point on a centimeter scale at one third of the anteroposterior centimeter
   measurement of the patient.

   Tomographic exposures are taken posteriorly from the level at
   0.5 cm. levels to a depth of 2 cm.

   c) Target-film distance: 36 inches.

2. *Measurements*

   See Figure 212.

   Maximum width of the common duct is measured in the supra-ampullary
   portion.

MEASUREMENT OF COMMON BILE DUCT DIAMETER

COMMON DUCT SIZE

Normal:
    Average diameter (mm.) 5.5
    Range (mm.) 3-9
Diameter greater than 10 mm. is abnormal.

Postcholecystectomy:
    Average diameter (mm.) 9
    Range (mm.) 3-30

3. *Source of Material*

Numerous articles have been published on the subject of common duct size. The measurements shown above have been selected as most representative; and, for further information, the reader is referred to the four articles listed below:

Anderson, F. G.: Am. J. Roentgenol. 78:623, 1957.

Beargie, R. J., *et al.:* Surg., Gynec. & Obst. 115:143, 1962.

Edmunds, R.; Rucker, C.; and Finby, N.: Arch. Surg. 90:73, 1965.

Wise, R. E.; Johnston, D. O.; and Salzman, F. A.: Radiology 68:507, 1957.

MEASUREMENT OF THE VELOCITY OF PORTAL VEIN BLOOD FLOW*

1. *Technique*

 a) Central ray: Centered over spleen.
 b) Position: Anteroposterior abdomen.
 c) Target-film distance: 100 cm.

 Films taken in deep inspiration.

 Thirty cc. of Triurol 50% (sodium acetrizoate: specific gravity 1.3; viscosity at 37° C., 2.1 centipoise) was injected into the spleen at the rate of 6-7.5 cc./sec. Films were taken with an automatic film changer at a rate of 1 film per second for 13 seconds after the beginning of the injection; then 1 film every 3 seconds for 20 seconds.

2. *Measurements*

 The velocity of flow was estimated in four ways:
 a) Measurement of the distance that the head of the contrast medium had advanced between two consecutive exposures was assessed in centimeters per second.
 b) Spleen-hilum time = Interval between the beginning of the injection of contrast medium and the demonstration of the bifurcation of the portal trunk in the liver hilum.
 c) Spleen-liver time = Interval between the beginning of injection of contrast medium in the smallest observable intrahepatic portal branches in the right liver lobe.
 d) Emptying time of the portal branches = Interval between the end of the injection and the moment that the intrahepatic portal branches are no longer discernible.

 The portal vein blood flow data are summarized in the following chart:

METHOD	RANGE	MEAN	IN NORMAL CONTROLS	IN PATIENTS WITH PORTAL HYPERTENSION
Velocity (cm./sec.)	8-42	21.6	15 or more	15 or less[†]
Spleen-hilum time (sec.)	½-3	1.7	2 or less	2 or more
Spleen-liver time (sec.)	3-6	4.3	5 or less	5+
Emptying time of portal branches (sec.)	3-7	4.3	5 or less	5+

 [†]On one half of the patients

3. *Source of Material*

 Sixteen adults with normal circulation in the portal system were compared with 54 patients with portal hypertension.

 Note:

 Average linear velocity of portal vein flow ranged from 15.5 to 24.1 cm./sec. in 6 patients studied by Sovak and others. (Sovak, M.; Soulen, R. L.; and Reichle, F. A.: Radiology 99:531, 1971.)

---

*Bergstrand, I., and Eckman, C.-A.: Acta radiol. 47:1, 1957.

MEASUREMENT OF THE DUODENAL MAJOR PAPILLA OF VATER*

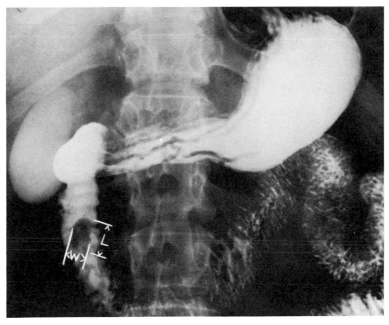

FIG. 213.

1. Technique

a) Central ray: To 2d lumbar vertebra.

b) Position: Posteroanterior abdomen for stomach and duodenum.

c) Target-film distance: 36 inches.

2. Measurements

See Figure 213.

Measurements of major papilla from anatomic specimens:

	LENGTH	WIDTH	HEIGHT
Average size (cm.)	1.5	0.5	0.5
Minimum size (cm.)...........	0.1	0.1	0.1
Maximum size (cm.)	3.0	1.2	1.2

Measurements from series of gastrointestinal films:

	LENGTH *(L)*	WIDTH *(W)*
Average size (cm.)	1.5	0.7

The papilla position is most frequently on the medial duodenal wall toward the posterior portion of the middescending duodenum.

3. Source of Material

The anatomic measurements were made on 100 specimens described as normal, fresh, and unassociated with any history, symptoms, or gross evidence of disease referable to the biliary tract, pancreas, or duodenum.

The measurements of papilla size from the films correspond well to the anatomic measurements.

---

*Poppel, M. H.; Jacobsen, H. G.; and Smith, R. W.: *The Roentgen Aspects of the Papilla and Ampulla of Vater* (Springfield, Ill.: Charles C Thomas, Publisher, 1953).

SMALL BOWEL CALIBER IN CHILDREN AND ADULTS*

1. Technique

    a) Central ray: Perpendicular to plane of film centered over midabdomen.

    b) Position: Anteroposterior with patient supine.

    c) Target-film distance: Children—36 inches.

                          Adults—30 inches.

2 Measurements

Nonflocculating media which are complex barium sulphate suspensions are used. A 50% dilution in volume of 2 to 8 oz. is used according to age in children and according to size of stomach in adults. Three segments of the small bowel which have clearly defined margins and approximately the same caliber as the rest of the small bowel are selected for measurement. The measurements are made at right angles to the parallel margins of the bowel. The average of the three measurements is used.

MEAN DIAMETER OF SMALL BOWEL

Age	Diameter (mm.) 1 S.D. = 1.9 mm.
6 mos.	12.0
1 yr.	13.0
2 yrs.	15.0
3 yrs.	16.7
4 yrs.	18.9
5 yrs.	19.0
6 yrs.	19.9
7 yrs.	20.5
8 yrs.	21.0
9 yrs.	21.4
10 yrs.	21.8
11 yrs.	22.1
12 yrs.	22.3
13 yrs.	22.5
14 yrs.	22.7
15 yrs.	23.0

Adult value is 23.1 mm. ± 1.9 (1 S.D.). Upper limit for adult is 25 mm.

(From Haworth *et al.*, Table 2.)

3. Source of Material

Small bowel measurements were taken from 61 infants and children aged 9 months to 15½ years and from 77 adults (37 males and 40 females) aged 19 to 77 years.

---

*Haworth, E. M.; Hodson, C. J.; Joyce, R. B.; *et al.:* Clin. Radiol. 18:417, 1967. (By kind permission of the honorary editor of Clinical Radiology.)

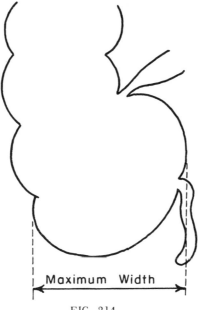

Maximum Width

FIG. 214.

1. *Technique*

   a) Central ray: On median plane at level of iliac crests.
   b) Position: Posteroanterior.
   c) Target-film distance: 36 inches.

2. *Measurements*

   See Figure 214.

   The greatest transverse diameter is measured on the prone film of the abdomen.
   Average diameter = 5-7 cm.

   A width of 9 cm. or greater is a critical diameter beyond which danger of perforation exists.

3. *Source of Material*

   Artificial distention of the cecum with barium and air was performed on 100 selected patients without intrinsic cecal disease or distal large bowel obstruction. Nineteen cases of cecal distention with distal large-bowel obstruction were studied for comparison.

*Davis, L., and Lowman, R. M.: Radiology 68:542, 1957.

MEASUREMENT OF THE ILEOCECAL VALVE*

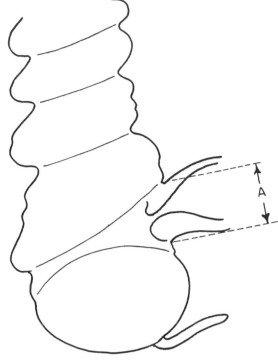

FIG. 215.

1. *Technique*

   a) Central ray: Spot roentgenograms made during fluoroscopy.

   b) Position: Posterior and oblique views (found to best demonstrate the valve during fluoroscopy), using graduated pressure over ileocecal valve region.

   c) Target-film distance: Depends on patient thickness.

2. *Measurements*

   See Figure 215.

   Average vertical diameter *(A)* = 2.5 cm.

   Vertical diameter *(A)* of 4.0 cm. or more is considered abnormal by Hinkel.

3. *Source of Measurement*

   Five hundred consecutive routine barium enema examinations.

*Hinkel, C. L.: Am. J. Roentgenol. 68:171, 1952.

MEASUREMENT OF THE PRESACRAL SPACE
IN CHILDREN* AND ADULTS†

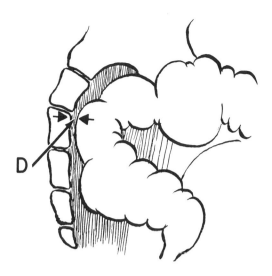

FIG. 216.

1. *Technique*

   a) Central ray: Spot roentgenograms made during fluoroscopy.
   b) Position: Lateral view obtained during barium enema examination.
   c) Target-film distance: Variable; depends on width of patient.

2. *Measurements*

   See Figure 216.
   The shortest distance between the posterior rectum and the sacrum is indicated by *D*.

   > *Children* (ages 1 to 15 years)
   > Distance (*D*): Average 3 mm.
   >   Range 1-5 mm.
   > Measurements over 5 mm. should be considered abnormal.
   > *Adults*†
   > Distance (*D*): Average 7 mm.
   >   Range 2-16 mm.
   > Measurements over 20 mm. should be considered abnormal.

3. *Source of Material*

   Eklöf and Gierup studied 85 boys and 75 girls in the 1-to-15-year age group who had no evidence of inflammatory bowel disease.
   Chrispin and Fry studied 100 patients, selected at random, in whom no bowel abnormality could be demonstrated.

*Eklöf, O., and Gierup, J.: Am. J. Roentgenol. 108:624, 1970.

†Chrispin, A. R., and Fry, I. K.: Brit. J. Radiol. 36:319, 1963.

243

VII. THE SPLEEN AND ADRENAL GLANDS

MEASUREMENT OF SPLEEN POSITION AND SIZE*

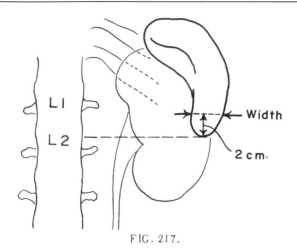

FIG. 217.

1. *Technique*

   a) Central ray: At level of iliac crests on median plane.

   b) Position: Anteroposterior.

   c) Target-film distance: 36 inches.

2. *Measurements*

   See Figure 217.

   The transverse diameter of the lower pole of the spleen was determined at a point 2 cm. above the tip of the lower pole.

NO. OF CASES	AGE (YEARS)	LEVEL OF LOWER POLE TIP	WIDTH (IN CM.) AT 2 CM. ABOVE TIP OF SPLEEN
16	Under 5	L1-L3 (usually L2)	2.0-3.6 (av., 3.0)
37	5-10	L1-L3 (usually L1-L2)	2.5-3.8 (av., 3.3)
36	11-20	L1-L3 (usually L1-L2)	2.5-3.8 (av., 3.2)
82	21-30	T12-L2 (usually L1)	2.0-4.2 (av., 3.5)
117	Over 30	T12-L2 (usually L1)	2.0-4.6 (av., 3.5)

Total 288

Enlargement of the splenic shadow occurs in a significantly large number of cases of ruptured spleen. Since the spleen outline is not demonstrated in 58% of abdominal roentgenograms, absence of this sign does not exclude the diagnosis of ruptured spleen.

3. *Source of Material*

   Five hundred consecutive cases with films of the abdomen were evaluated regardless of the diagnostic problem.

*Wyman, A. C.: Am. J. Roentgenol. 72:51, 1954.

MEASUREMENT OF SPLEEN LENGTH*

1. *Technique*

   a) Central ray: Centered over spleen.
   b) Position: Anteroposterior abdomen.
   c) Target-film distance: 100 cm.

   Film taken in deep inspiration.

2. *Measurements*

   The spleen length is the distance between the level of the most cranial part of the diaphragmatic arch and the lower pole of the spleen.
   Mean length = 12.4 ± 2.2 cm. (range, 8-19 cm.).
   If the spleen length exceeds 16 cm., there is 97% probability that the spleen is enlarged.

3. *Source of Material*

   Studies were made of 50 adults (23 men, 27 women) without known symptoms or signs of liver or spleen disease.

DETERMINATION OF SPLEEN MASS FROM RADIONUCLIDE IMAGES

A method of estimating spleen mass from posterior and left lateral views of the radionuclide photoscans is described in the following articles:

Rollo, F. D., and De Land, F. H.: Radiology 97:583, 1970.
De Land, F. H.: Radiology 97:589, 1970.

---

*Bergstrand, I., and Ekman, C.-A.: Acta Radiol. 47:1, 1957.

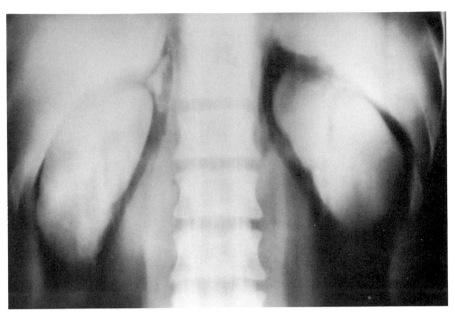

FIG. 218.—Normal extraperitoneal pneumogram. The right adrenal is triangular, and the left semilunar. (Steinbach and Smith, Fig. 1.)

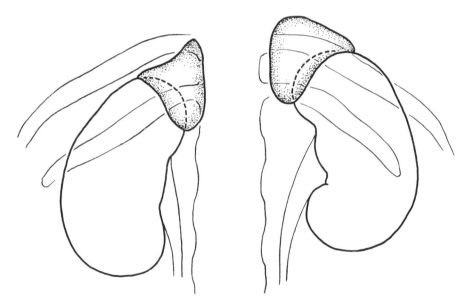

FIG. 219.—Diagram to illustrate shape of adrenal glands.

*Steinbach, H. L., and Smith, D. R.: A.M.A. Arch. Surg. 70:161, 1955.

MEASUREMENT OF ADRENAL GLAND SIZE

1. *Technique*

   a) Central ray: At level of iliac crests on median plane.

   b) Position: Anteroposterior abdomen.

   c) Target-film distance: 40 inches.

2. *Measurements*

   See Figures 218 and 219.

   The cross-sectional area of the gland was obtained by tracing the gland contour with a compensating planimeter. The same results may be obtained by tracing the contour of the gland on 1 mm. graph paper and counting the enclosed squares.

   AVERAGE ADRENAL CROSS-SECTIONAL AREA

   Right .... 4.2 cm.^{2}

   Left...................................... 4.3 cm.^{2}

   Range—right .... 2.0 - 7.8 cm.^{2}

   Range—left .... 2.0 - 8.7 cm.^{2}

   Holmes, Moon, and Rinehart* have shown that the weight of the adrenal is related to body weight and surface area. The weight of adrenals in males was greater than in females by 11%; but when the figures were corrected for body size, the females had slightly more adrenal tissue per kilogram of body weight or square centimeter of body surface than the males.

3. *Source of Material*

   Study of 25 normal adults.

---

*Holmes, R. O.; Moon, H. D.; and Rinehart, J. F.: Am. J. Path. 27:724, 1951.

VIII. THE URINARY TRACT

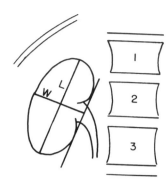

FIG. 220.—(From Friedenberg, Fig. 1.)

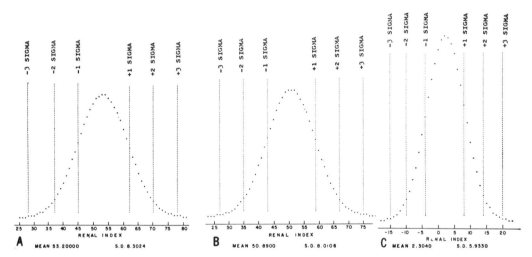

A   MEAN 53.20000   S.D. 8.3024

B   MEAN 50.8900   S.D. 8.0106

C   MEAN 2.3040   S.D. 5.9330

Graph IA.   Left renal index—children.   Frequency plot of theoretical normal distribution.
Graph IB.   Right renal index—children.   Frequency plot of theoretical normal distribution.
Graph IC.   Left minus right renal index—children.   Frequency plot of theoretical normal distribution.

Graphs IA-IC, IIA-IIC, and IIIA-IIIC from Friedenberg.)

*Friedenberg, M. J., et al.: Radiology 84: 1022, 1965.

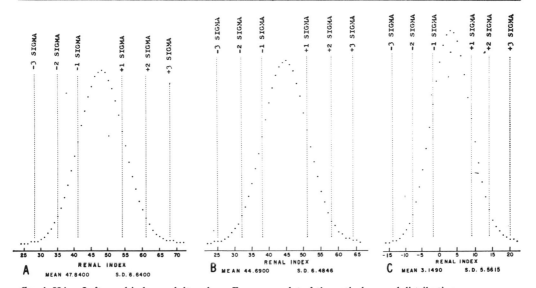

Graph IIA.   Left renal index—adult males.   Frequency plot of theoretical normal distribution.
Graph IIB.   Right renal index—adult males.   Frequency plot of theoretical normal distribution.
Graph IIC.   Left minus right renal index—adult males.   Frequency plot of theoretical normal distribution.

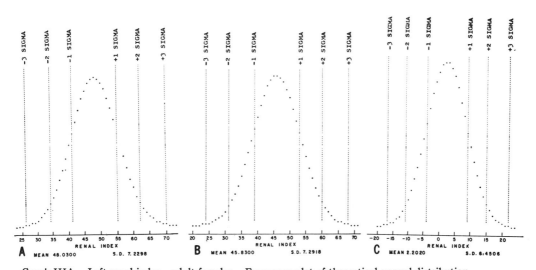

Graph IIIA.   Left renal index—adult females.   Frequency plot of theoretical normal distribution.
Graph IIIB.   Right renal index—adult females.   Frequency plot of theoretical normal distribution.
Graph IIIC.   Left minus right renal index—adult females.   Frequency plot of theoretical normal distribution.

253

1. *Technique*

   a) Central ray: Centered over midabdomen.
   b) Position: Anteroposterior with patient supine.
   c) Target-film distance: 40 inches.

2. *Measurements*

   See Figure 220.

   The length of each kidney was determined by measuring the maximum distance from the cephalad to the caudad margin. The medial margin was determined by drawing a line between the most medial aspects of the upper and lower poles. The width was then ascertained by measuring the maximum distance from the lateral to the medial margin along a line perpendicular to the length line. The body surface area of each patient was obtained from his height and weight by use of the DuBois nomogram (pp. 200 and 202). A renal index was calculated for each kidney, defined according to the following formula:

   $$RI = \frac{L \times W}{BSA}$$

   where RI is the renal index, L is the length of the kidney in centimeters, W is the width of the kidney in centimeters, and BSA is the body surface area of the patient in square meters. The values obtained and the left *minus* the right renal indices are given in the graphs (Graph IA-IIIC) following Figure 220.

   (See pp. 255-257 for alternate approaches to this measurement.)

3. *Source of Material*

   The data are based on a study of 1,286 people, Caucasian and Negro (322 children, 363 male adults, and 601 female adults), from the general population of a large hospital. These individuals had extensive renal disease, as determined by history, physical examination, and routine laboratory findings.

A. In Children

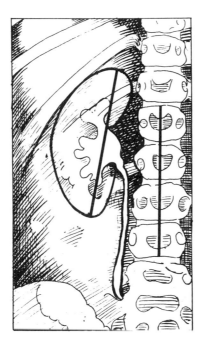

FIG. 221.—(From Currarino, Fig. 3.*)

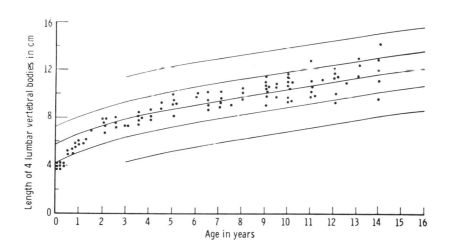

Length of the four lumbar vertebral bodies superimposed on the graph for kidney length.
(From Currarino, Fig. 4.*)

*Currarino, G.: Am. J. Roentgenol. 93:464, 1965.

SIZE OF NORMAL KIDNEYS RELATED TO VERTEBRAL HEIGHT

A. In Children

1. Technique

a) Central ray: Perpendicular to plane of film centered over midabdomen.

b) Position: Anteroposterior with patient supine.

c) Target-film distance: Immaterial.

2. Measurements

See Figure 221.

The maximum length of the kidney and the length of the first four lumbar vertebral bodies, including the three intervertebral spaces comprised by them, are measured as shown in Figure 221. The values obtained were plotted against age; and the results were superimposed on the graph for kidney length, as shown in Figure 221. The length of this segment of the lumbar spine corresponded to the normal length of the kidney (± 1 cm.) throughout childhood with the exception of the first $1\frac{1}{2}$ years of life, in which the length of a normal kidney was greater. A difference in length of the two kidneys up to 1 cm. can occur normally.

3. Source of Material

The data were derived from a review of excretory urograms of 50 children from 0 to 14 years. Males and females were represented in nearly equal numbers. All children had no evidence of urinary tract disease. The vertebral measurements were made in this group as well as in 50 normal unselected children 0-14 years of age.

Note:

C. J. Hodson (Radiology 88:857, 1967) has shown a linear relationship between kidney length and body height in children.

B. In Adults

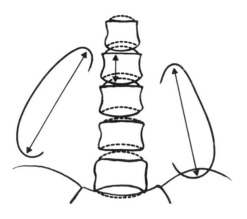

FIG. 222.—(Redrawn from Simon.)

Age (dec-ade)	Mean Weight (gm.)	Mean Length (cm.)	Mean Ratio (kidney length/ height of L2)	Mean Ratio (kidney length/ height of L2 plus disk)
2nd	210	12.4	4.1	3.6
3rd	170	12.2	3.5	3.0
4th	155	11.2	3.5	3.0
5th	135	12.2	3.8	3.1
6th	145	11.8	3.7	3.1
7th	125	11.5	3.6	3.1
8th	120	11.3	3'.7	3.1
9th	100	11.4	3.7	3.1

(From Simon, Table 2.)

*Simon, A. L.: Am. J. Roentgenol: 92:270, 1964.

B. In Adults

1. *Technique*

a) Central ray: Perpendicular to plane of film centered over midabdomen.
b) Position: Anteroposterior supine.
c) Target-film distance: Immaterial.

2. *Measurements*

See Figure 222.

The length of each kidney was determined in its longest axis. The height of the 2d lumbar vertebral body was determined with and without the L2-L3 disk. The measurements were made at the posterior margins of the body. These are then used to create two sets of ratios: kidney length/height of L2 and kidney length/height of L2 plus disk. The normal values are given in the table accompanying Figure 222.

3. *Source of Material*

The data were derived from a study of roentgenograms of 100 consecutive patients with autopsy-proved kidneys of normal weight and normal gross and microscopic appearance. There were 55 females and 45 males, ranging in age from 23 to 86 years. About half of the patients were in the sixth and seventh decades.

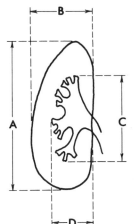

FIG. 223.—(Redrawn from Vuorinen *et al.*, Fig. 1.)

1. *Technique*

a) Central ray: Perpendicular to plane of film centered over midabdomen.

b) Position: Anteroposterior supine.

c) Target-film distance: Immaterial.

2. *Measurements*

See Figure 223.

The upper and lower poles are marked. The lateral and medial borders are marked. The renal calyceal system is outlined and the superior, inferior and lateral calyces are marked. The distances between the marked lines are measured in millimeters.

$$\text{Renal Cortical Index } (RCI) = \frac{C \text{ (mm.)} \times D \text{ (mm.)}}{A \text{ (mm.)} \times B \text{ (mm.)}}$$

RCI (mean value of both kidneys of a patient) = 0.35; S.D. = 0.04.

RCI/D is the difference in *RCI* between the two kidneys of the same patient = 0.02; S.D. = 0.02.

3. *Source of Material*

One hundred six normal patients.

*Vuorinen, P.; Anttila, P.; Wegelius, U.; *et al.*: Acta radiol. supp. 211, 1962.

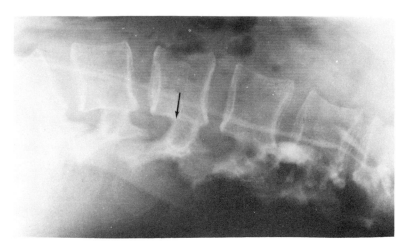

FIG. 224.–(From Cook *et al.*, Fig. 1.)

1. Technique

    a) Central ray: Perpendicular to plane of film centered to lateral midabdomen in cross-table lateral projection.

    b) Position: Patient supine. Cross-table lateral.

    c) Target-film distance: 40 inches.

2. Measurements

    See Figure 224.

    Measure the distance from the posterior margin of the renal pelvis to the midpoint of the posterior surface of the adjacent vertebral body.

DISTANCE OF THE POSTERIOR MARGIN OF THE RENAL PELVIS FROM THE POSTERIOR SURFACE OF THE ADJACENT VERTEBRAL BODY

Vertebral Level	No. of Renal Pelves	Mean Distance (mm.)	Standard Deviation
D-12	7	1.6	8.2
L-1	79	8.6	9.7
L-2	91	9.0	8.8
L-3	6	–1.00	5.9

(From Cook *et al.*, Table 1.)

*Cook, I. K.; Keats, T. E.; and Seale, D. L.: Radiology 99:499, 1971.

NORMAL POSITION OF RENAL PELVES AND
URETERS ON THE LATERAL UROGRAM

DISTANCE OF THE POSTERIOR MARGIN OF THE URETER FROM THE POSTERIOR SURFACE OF THE ADJACENT VERTEBRAL BODY

Vertebral Level	No. of Ureters	Mean Distance (mm.)	Standard Deviation	Distances That Would Occur <1% of the Time (mm.)
L-1	4	16.8	7.4	33.0
L-2	54	24.2	9.3	45.9
L-3	116	29.7	10.1	53.2
L-4	116	38.8	9.7	61.4
L-5	116	49.2	9.5	71.3

(From Cook *et al.*, Table 2.)

DISTANCE OF THE POSTERIOR MARGIN OF THE URETER FROM THE POSTERIOR SURFACE OF THE ADJACENT VERTEBRAL BODY EXPRESSED IN VERTEBRAL WIDTHS

Vertebral Level	No. of Ureters	Mean Vertebral Width	Standard Deviation
L-3	116	0.75	0.23
L-4	116	0.99	0.20
L-5	116	1.25	0.31

(From Cook *et al.*, Table 3.)

3. Source of Material

One hundred five patients with normal excretory urograms. Thirty-five were men and 70 were women. Ages ranged from 14 to 76 years.

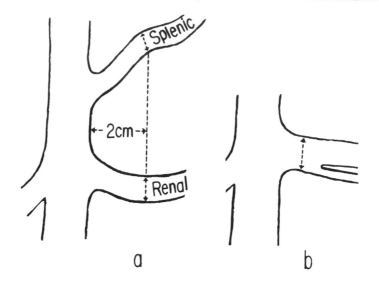

FIG. 225.—(Redrawn from Maluf.)

INTERNAL DIAMETER OF RENAL ARTERY

		S.D.
Two normal kidneys	6.5 — 6.7 mm.	0.75 — 0.88
One healthy hyper-trophied kidney	8.4 — 8.6 mm.	0.71 — 0.83

$$\text{Normal ratio:} \quad \frac{\text{Diameter of renal artery}}{\text{Splenic artery}} = \; > 1$$

*Maluf, N. S. R.: Surg., Gynec. & Obst. 107:415, 1958.

MEASUREMENT OF RENAL ARTERY SIZE

1. *Technique*

   a) Central ray: Perpendicular to plane of film centered over the interspace between the 1st and 2d lumbar vertebral bodies.

   b) Position: Anteroposterior.

   c) Target-film distance: 32 inches. Measurements are reduced by 10% for distortion.

2. *Measurements*

   See Figure 225.

   a) The renal and splenic arteries are measured where they intersect a line 2 cm. from and parallel to the lateral border of the aorta. The measurements are made at right angles to the longitudinal axis of the vessel at the 2 cm. intersection.

   b) When the renal artery bifurcates at a point closer than 2 cm. from the aorta, it is measured proximal to this bifurcation. When a kidney receives more than one artery from the aorta, the equivalent diameter *(D)* is obtained from the equation:

   $$D = 4\sqrt{D_1^4 + D_2^4 + \ldots D_n^4}$$

   in which D_1 and D_2 are the diameters of two such arteries and D_n the diameter of the nth such artery.

   Of greater value is the ratio of internal diameter of the renal artery to the splenic artery. This is typically greater than unity when the kidney is normal. The ratio rises in renal hypertrophy and falls in renal hypoplasia or reduced renal function. A narrow renal artery is always indicative of reduced renal function, but an artery of normal caliber does not necessarily imply normal renal function.

3. *Source of Material*

   The data are based on measurements of 18 young patients with normal kidneys, 9 young patients with only one healthy hypertrophied kidney, and 32 patients with unilateral or bilateral renal abnormality.

RELATIONSHIP OF RENAL SURFACE AND
PARENCHYMA AREAS TO RENAL ARTERY SIZE*

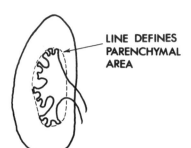

LINE DEFINES
PARENCHYMAL
AREA

FIG. 226.—(From Wojtowicz, Fig. 1.)

1. Technique

a) Central ray: Perpendicular to plane of film centered over the interspace between the 1st and 2nd lumbar vertebral bodies.

b) Position: Anteroposterior.

c) Target-film distance: 95 cm.

2. Measurements

See Figure 226.

Study performed using selective renal or abdominal aortography. Serial angiographic films and urographic films were obtained in moderate inspiration. Measurements made as follows:

a) Renal area is determined with a planimeter from the nephrographic phase.

b) Renal parenchyma area is defined by a line drawn through the calyceal fornices and the intrarenal part of the renal pelvis. The parenchymal area is calculated as the difference between the renal area and the area of the pyelocalyceal system.

c) Renal artery diameter is measured at a distance 1 cm. from the origin of the artery. Cross-sectional area of the artery is expressed as the square of the artery radius (the constant π is omitted).

*Wojtowicz, J.: Invest. Radiol. 2:231, 1967.

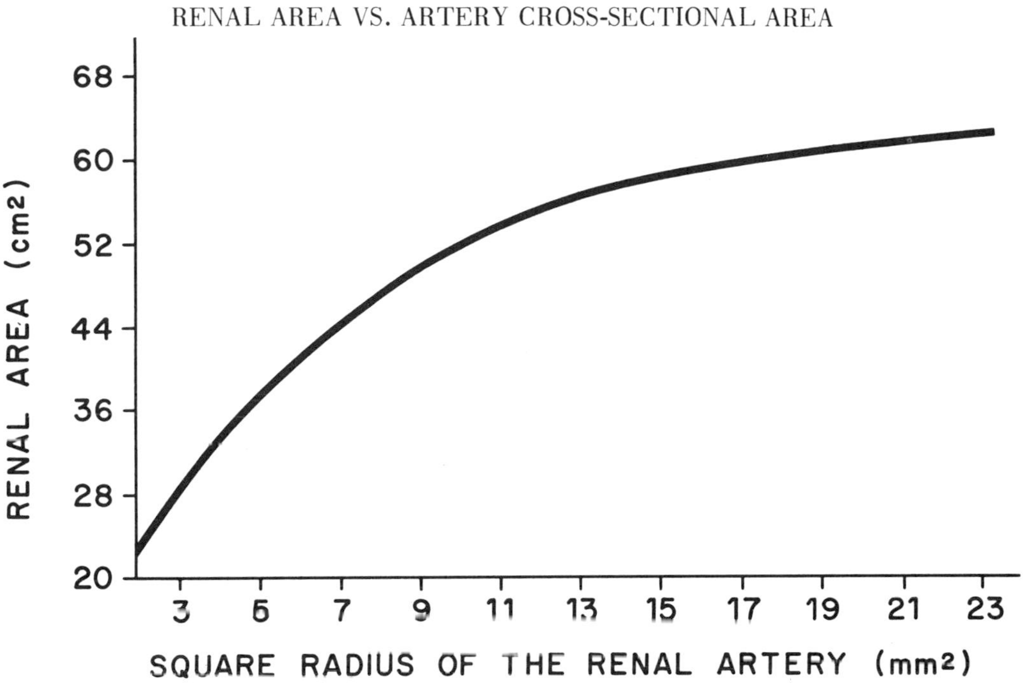

RELATIONSHIP OF RENAL SURFACE AND
PARENCHYMA AREAS TO RENAL ARTERY SIZE

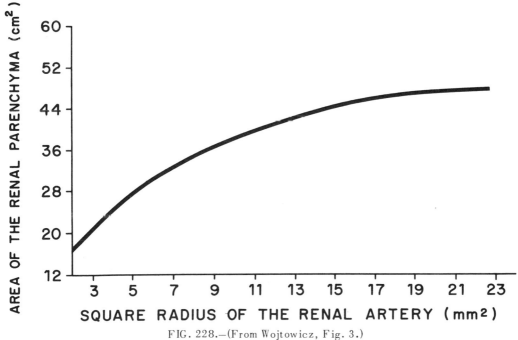

RENAL AREA VS. ARTERY CROSS-SECTIONAL AREA

FIG. 227.—(From Wojtowicz, Fig. 2.)

RENAL PARENCHYMA AREA VS. ARTERY CROSS-SECTION AREA

FIG. 228.—(From Wojtowicz, Fig. 3.)

3. Source of Material

One hundred twenty-four renal angiograms in patients with a single arterial blood supply to each kidney. Some selected cases with pathology were included.

MEASUREMENT OF THE URETHROVESICAL ANGLES IN STRESS INCONTINENCE

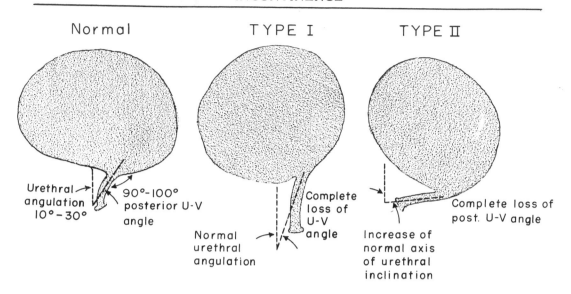

Normal   TYPE I   TYPE II

Urethral angulation 10°–30°

90°–100° posterior U-V angle

Normal urethral angulation

Complete loss of U-V angle

Increase of normal axis of urethral inclination

Complete loss of post. U-V angle

(Modified from T.H. Green*.)

1. *Technique*

a) Central ray: At level of greater trochanter perpendicular to plane of film.
b) Position: Lateral erect straining.
c) Target-film distance: Immaterial.

2. *Measurements*

Angles are determined by chain cystourethrography in the erect position during straining. The angle between the posterior aspect of the urethra and the base of the bladder (posterior urethrovesical angle) normally measures 90°–100°. Loss of this angle alone indicates Type I stress incontinence. The angle of inclination of the urethra is found by extending a line through the direction of the upper urethra to join a line in the vertical axis of the patient. The normal angle is 10° to 30° and an angle above 45° is definitely abnormal. Loss of this angle plus loss of the posterior urethral angle constitutes Type II stress incontinence.

3. *Source of Material*

The data on the posterior urethrovesical angle is based on a study of more than 500 roentgen examinations of the bladder and urethra of 132 non-pregnant women.[†]
The data on the angle of inclination of the urethra is based on a study of 350 patients examined by cystourethrography.[‡]

Green* notes that angle measurements do not apply if a cystocele is present. The chain cystourethrogram is usually abnormal in stress incontinence. However, an abnormal cystourethrogram does not necessarily indicate stress incontinence.

*Green, T.H., Jr.: Am. J. Obst. & Gynec. 83:632, 1962.

†Jeffcoate, T.N.A., and Roberts, H.: J. Obst. & Gynaec. Brit. Emp. 59:685, 1952.

‡Bailey, K.V.: J. Obst. & Gynaec. Brit. Emp. 63:663, 1956.

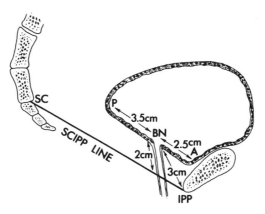

FIG. 229.—Composite drawing of lateral recumbent film showing average normal adult female measurements. (From Noll and Hutch, Fig. 12.)

1. Technique

a) Central ray: At level of greater trochanter perpendicular to plane of film.

b) Positions: Lateral recumbent.

Lateral erect straining.

Lateral erect voiding.

c) Target-film distance: 36 inches.

2. Measurements

See Figure 229.

The bladder is filled with opaque medium until the patient experiences discomfort. A small chain of metal beads is used to demonstrate the urethrovesical angle. A line (SCIPP) is drawn from the sacrococcygeal joint *(SC)* to the inferior point of the pubic bone *(IPP)*. *BN* is the bladder neck, and the flat base of the bladder is the base plate.

Average measurements (cm.) in lateral recumbent position:

	Average (cm.)
Base plate: Range 5-7 cm.	6.0
Base plate: Anterior to bladder neck	2.5
Base plate: Posterior to bladder neck	3.5
Bladder neck above SCIPP line	2.0
Bladder neck to *IPP*	3.0

In standing position the bladder neck drops 1 cm. from recumbent position.

In standing position with straining the bladder neck drops an additional 1 cm, or 2 cm. compared with recumbent.

In standing position with voiding the bladder neck drops an additional 0.5 cm. to 2.5 cm. compared with recumbent.

*Noll, L. E., and Hutch, J. A.: Obst. & Gynec. 33:680, 1969.

THE SACROCOCCYGEAL – INFERIOR PUBIC POINT (SCIPP)
LINE AND THE LATERAL CYSTOURETHROGRAM

In patients with stress incontinence the recumbent film showed a rounded base plate for about one half of the patients. The bladder neck averaged 1 cm. above the SCIPP line. The drop in the bladder neck upon standing, straining and voiding was greater in distance than for the normal group.

3. Source of Material

Ninety-five adult women, of whom 20 were urologically normal.

Note:

A data sheet has been designed by Noll and Hutch (*op. cit.*, Fig. 11) which enables the radiologist to record readily all pertinent cystourethrogram information.

MEASUREMENT OF THE URETHRA IN CHILDREN*

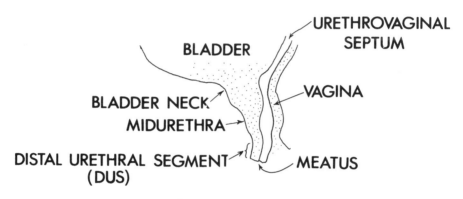

FIG. 230.—(Redrawn from Shopfner, Fig. 1.)

1. Technique

- *a)* Central ray: Television fluoroscopy and spot roentgenograms made during the voiding cycle.
- *b)* Position: Oblique and lateral views obtained during voiding cystourethrography.
- *c)* Target-film distance: Variable; Shopfner used a 15% correction for magnification.

2. Measurements

See Figure 230.

For females the meatus was indicated by barium coating of the mucosa or by identification of the urethrovaginal septum. Diameters of meatus, distal urethral segment (DUS) and midurethra were measured on films taken during full voiding.

For males the urethra was measured at the midpart of the membranous and the posterior urethra.

---

*Shopfner, C. E.: Radiology 88:222, 1967.

MEASUREMENT OF THE URETHRA IN CHILDREN

URETHROGRAM MEASUREMENTS (PERCENTAGE OF PATIENTS)

Diameters (mm.)	Females			Males	
	Meatus %	DUS %	Midurethra %	Membranous Urethra %	Posterior Urethra %
2	4	4		4	
3	16	16		8	
4	20	20	1	16	1
5	31	28	3	26	5
6	25	21	9	24	8
7	4	9	11	16	18
8		2	25	4	24
9			12	2	11
10			4		13
11			5		3
12			17		4
13			4		4
14			1.5		1
15			2		2
16			2		1
17			0.05		1
18			1		1
19			1		1
20			0.05		1
21			0.05		1

Measurements made during full voiding stream.

(From Shopfner, Table 2.)

3. Source of Material

Fifty-three females and 67 males with no urinary-tract abnormality. Ages ranged from less than 1 year to 16 years.

IX. PELVIMETRY AND FETOMETRY

MEASUREMENT OF THE PELVIS AND THE FETAL CRANIUM

From the many methods of roentgenographic measurement of the pelvis, two were chosen for presentation. One, the Ball method, employs geometric corrections based on target-film and object-film distances; the other, the Colcher-Sussman method, makes corrections by comparing measured diameters with a centimeter scale placed at the same distance from the film as the internal diameters to be measured and projected on the same film.

As Maloy and Swenson* state, "One method is probably as accurate as another if done with the precision advocated by its author. Each radiologist should select a method and learn to use it well, bearing constantly in mind the importance of the shape of the pelvis, which is not necessarily reflected in the measurements of the cardinal diameters alone."

A. The Ball Method†

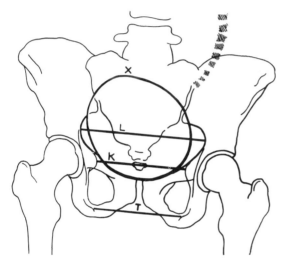

FIG. 231.—Anteroposterior view of pelvis made near term. (From Maloy and Swenson, Fig. 102.)

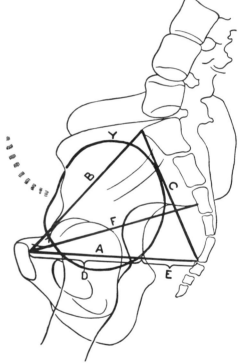

FIG. 232.—Lateral view of pelvis made near term with patient in erect position. (From Maloy and Swenson, Fig. 100.)

*Maloy, H. C., and Swenson, P. C.: *Diagnostic Roentgenology* (Ross Golden, ed.), Vol. 2 (Baltimore: Williams & Wilkins Company, 1952).

†Ball, R. P., and Golden, R.: Am. J. Roentgenol. 49:731, 1943.

MEASUREMENT OF THE PELVIS AND THE FETAL CRANIUM

A. The Ball Method

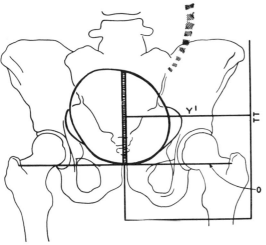

FIG. 233.—The object-film distance is one half the true bitrochanteric measurement of the patient plus the distance from table top to film (about 4 cm.). The true bitrochanteric measurement is equal to the distance between the mesial margins of the greater trochanters, 0, plus 4 cm. for a 36 inch target-film distance, or plus 2 cm. for a 30 inch target-film distance. Y' extends from the equatorial zone of the fetal cranium (as seen in Figure 232) to the table top. (From Ball and Golden, Fig. 8, and Maloy and Swenson, Fig. 103.)

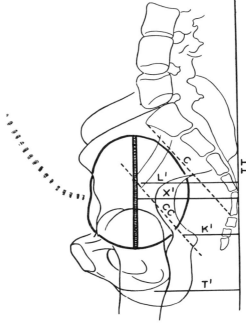

FIG. 234.—Object-table-top distances are represented by prime letters. Add approximately 4 cm. to obtain object-film distance. Line TT passes through the most posterior border of the sacrum and parallel to the film edge. The anterior point of L' is where a line CC, projected through the ischial spines and parallel to C, intersects the iliopectineal lines of the pelvic brim. The line K' extends from the ischial spine to table top, TT. The anterior point of T' lies in a vertical plane which intersects the inferior angles of the obturator foramina. The anterior point X' is the equatorial zone of the fetal cranium as seen on anteroposterior view (Fig. 233). (From Ball and Golden, Fig. 7, and Maloy and Swenson, Fig. 105.)

1. Technique

a) Central ray: Lateral, erect—To 1 inch above the superior margin of the greater trochanter. The central ray should pass through the posterosuperior margin of the greater trochanter. If the centering is correct, the sacroiliac notch shadows will be superimposed.

Anteroposterior, erect—To the median plane of the pelvis. Tube is moved upward 3 inches from the level used for the lateral view.

A. The Ball Method

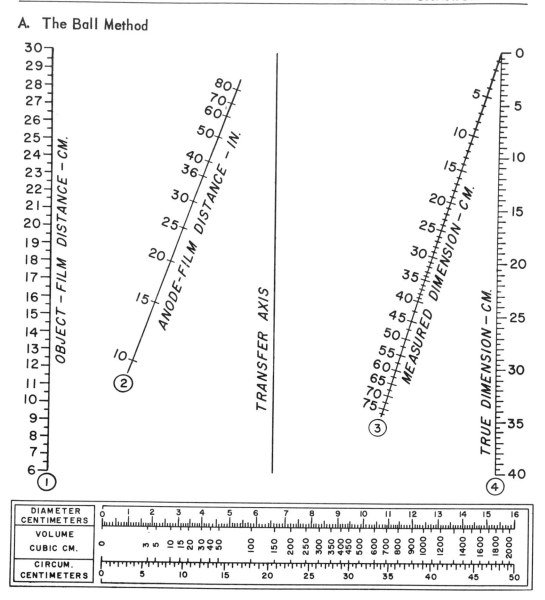

FIG. 235.—Nomogram (designed by Holmquist) for use with Ball method. Draw a straight line from the object-film distance *(1)* through the anode-film distance *(2)* to the transfer axis. Draw a second line from this point on the transfer axis through measured dimension *(3)* to true dimension *(4)*. Fetal skull volume can be found by using the circumference diameter scale at the bottom. (Adapted from Ball and Golden, Figs. 5 and 6.)

b) **Position:**   Lateral erect—The patient is placed in the lateral position with the right greater trochanter in contact with the surface of the erect Potter-Bucky diaphragm. Posterior curve of the sacrum falls about 1 inch anterior to posterior margin of the film. The inferior margin of the film should be at the level of the gluteal femoral crease.

           Anteroposterior, erect—The patient is positioned with her back to the Potter-Bucky diaphragm, and a compression band is applied.

c) **Target-film distance: 36 inches.**

MEASUREMENT OF THE PELVIS AND THE FETAL CRANIUM

A. The Ball Method

2. *Measurements*

   a) *Pelvis*

   Inlet: Anteroposterior diameter (promontory to pubis, Fig. 232,*B*) .... 11.5 cm.

   Widest transverse diameter (Fig. 231, *L*) .... 12.5 cm.

   Midpelvis: Anteroposterior diameter (pubic symphysis to lower end of 5th sacral segment, Fig. 232, *A*) .... 12.6 cm.

   This diameter is composed of two segments:

   The distance from pubic symphysis to interspinous plane (Fig. 232, *D)* .... 8.3 cm.

   The distance from interspinous plane to 5th sacral segment (Fig. 232, *E*) .... 4.3 cm.

   Interspinous diameter (Fig. 231, *K*)............................ 10.5 cm.

   Outlet: Transverse diameter (bituberal) (Fig. 231, *T*) .... 10.4 cm.

   b) *Fetal skull*

   The perimeter of the fetal skull outline on both the anteroposterior and lateral views is traced with a map measure, and each measurement is corrected for magnification. The two corrected measurements are averaged. This is the "mean circumference" of the skull. Two cm. is added to the mean circumference for the scalp thickness. This total circumference of the fetal head is translated into cubic centimeters (bottom scale, Fig. 235).

   The average mean circumference of fetal head (including the scalp), near term, equals 32.5-33.5 cm.

   The comparison between fetal head size and the smallest internal pelvic diameter is made by measuring certain of the pelvic dimensions. Most likely to cause trouble are the inlet anteroposterior diameter and the midplane interspinous diameter.

   The smallest of these two diameters and the total circumference of the fetal head are converted to cubic centimeters.

   When the volume of the fetal head is smaller than the volume of the largest sphere which could pass through the smallest dimension, no disproportion is present.

3. *Source of Material*

   Studies were made of 349 obstetrical patients examined in the Department of Radiology, Presbyterian Hospital, New York City.

A. The Ball Method: Friedman-Taylor Nomographic Aid*

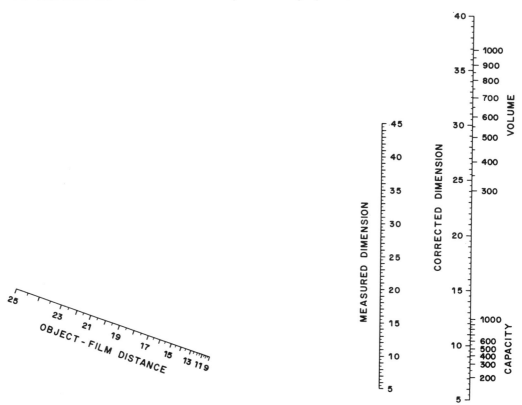

FIG. 236.—(From Friedman and Taylor, Fig. 3.)

1. Technique

a) Central ray: Use the Ball Method
b) Position: Use the Ball Method
c) Target-film distance: 40 inches. To use this nomogram (see Figure 236) you must use a target-film distance of 40 inches.

2. Measurements

Corrections of pelvic and fetal head measurements are made using appropriate object-film distances as follows:

a) Widest transverse diameter of the inlet (measured on anteroposterior film): Corrected using the distance from a point representing the widest diameter of the inlet (obtained by drawing a line parallel to the inclination of the sacrum through the ischial spines on the lateral x-ray view) to the posterior sacrum. To the latter measurement one should add an arbitrary figure of 4 cm. to take into account distance from the posterior bony aspect of the sacrum through the gluteal soft tissues to the film-holding cassette.

b) Interspinous diameter (measured on anteroposterior film): Corrected using distance from spine to posterior sacrum plus factor of 4 cm. (obtained from the lateral view).

c) Anteroposterior diameter of the inlet (measured on lateral view): Corrected by using distance from midpoint to greater trochanter plus 4 cm. (obtained from anteroposterior view).

*Friedman, E. A. and Taylor, M. B.: Am. J. Obst. & Gynec. 105:1110, 1969.

MEASUREMENT OF THE PELVIS AND THE FETAL CRANIUM

A. The Ball Method: Friedman-Taylor Nomographic Aid

d) Circumference of fetal head (measured on anteroposterior film): Corrected using distance from midpoint of head to posterior sacrum plus 4 cm. (obtained from lateral view).

e) Circumference of fetal head (measured on lateral view): Corrected using distance from midpoint to greater trochanter plus 4 cm. (obtained from anteroposterior view). If anteroposterior view head is not in midline, one uses the distance from midpoint of the fetal head to the appropriate greater trochanter. If the correct side is unknown, one measures to both trochanters independently and then uses only the measurement that approaches most closely that obtained after correcting the circumference of the anteroposterior view head.

The final step is the conversion of the corrected pelvic diameters to capacities and skull circumferences to volume. Comparison of capacities and volumes is made to evaluate the cephalopelvic relationship.

The following classification is useful:

a) *Inlet.* If inlet capacities are equal to or greater than fetal head volume, no disproportion exists. Cases in which the inlet capacities are smaller than the head volume by 50 cc. or less are deemed to have relative or borderline disproportion. Where the negative difference exceeds 50 cc. (head volume is more than 50 cc. larger than the smallest inlet capacity), "absolute" or high degree of disproportion is considered to be present.

b) *Midpelvis.* If the interspinous capacity is up to 150 cc. smaller than the volume of the head, no disproportion exists, between 150 and 200 cc. negative difference, there is relative midpelvic disproportion; if the negative difference exceeds 200 cc. at the midplane (head volume more than 200 cc. larger than interspinous capacity), interpretation of "absolute" disproportion is warranted.

3. Source of Measurements

Forty consecutive measurements of 5 pelvic and fetal skull dimensions.

B. The Colcher-Sussman Method*

POSITIONING

A

Lateral Positioning

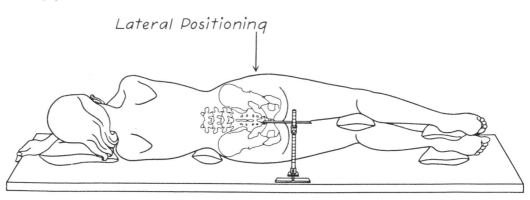

B

Antero Posterior Positioning

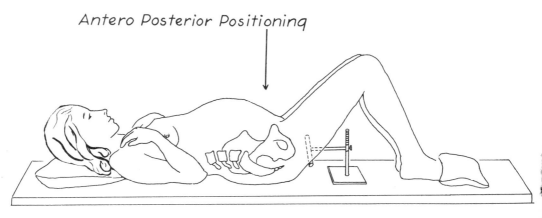

FIG. 237.–(From Colcher and Sussman, Fig. 3.)

Description of Intersecting Diameters (Fig. 238, *C* and *D*).

Inlet: Anteroposterior diameter *(I-G)*—Extends from upper inner margin of the symphysis to the interior surface of the sacrum following the level of the iliopectineal line, passing through a midpoint between the brim of the pelvis and the apices of the sacrosciatic notches. The apices of the notches must approximate each other.

Transverse diameter *(A-A')*—Widest transverse diameter of the inlet *(E)*.

Midpelvis: Anteroposterior diameter *(P-M)*—Extends from inner lower border of the pubic symphysis through the point halfway between the contours of the two ischial spines to the anterior margin of the sacrum.

Transverse diameter *(B-B')*—Transverse interspinous diameter *(F)*.

Outlet: Anteroposterior diameter (postsagittal, *S-T*)—Extends from the midbituberal point *(T)* to the lower anterior margin of the last sacral segment *(S)*.

*Colcher, A. E., and Sussman, W.: Am. J. Roentgenol. 51:207, 1944.

B. The Colcher-Sussman Method

POSITIONING WITH RULER

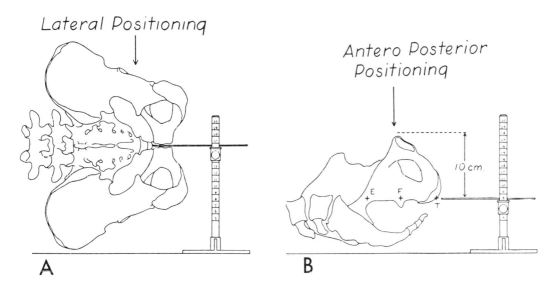

INTERSECTING DIAMETERS

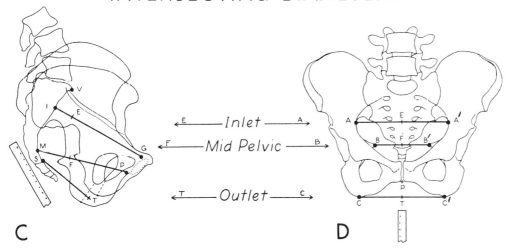

FIG. 232. (From Colcher and Sussman, Fig. 1.)

Point *T* is found as follows: On the lateral view, straight lines are projected from the lower border of each obturator foramen to the lowest point on the shadow of the ischial tuberosity. These lowest points (the bituberal points) are connected by a straight line. The midbituberal point *T* is halfway between these two points.

Transverse diameter (bituberal) *(C-C´)*—On the anteroposterior film, the points *C* and *C´* are obtained by projecting a straight line from the lateral margin of the inlet along the lateral wall of the forepelvis, which appears as a dense white line on the film to the lower margin of ischial tuberosity.

MEASUREMENT OF THE PELVIS AND THE FETAL CRANIUM

B. The Colcher-Sussman Method

1. Technique

a) Central ray: Lateral—To greater trochanter of femur.

Anteroposterior—To superior margin of pubic symphysis.

b) Positions: Lateral (Fig. 237, A)—True lateral with patient lying on either right or left side; knees and thighs semiflexed.

Anteroposterior (Fig. 237, B)—Patient supine with knees and thighs semiflexed and separated.

c) Target-film distance: 36 or 40 inches.

A specially devised ruler* is used to make measurement corrections. When positioned as described below, the ruler will have the same distortion as the diameters on the same level. Therefore, the ruler markings on the film become the centimeter scale.

Placement of ruler:

Lateral view (Fig. 237, A)—The ruler is placed at the midsacral spine parallel with the spine and film. The centimeter rule markings are projected on the film for direct mensuration.

Anteroposterior view (Fig. 237 B)—The ruler is placed at the level of the tuberosities of the ischium by direct manual palpation or by lowering the ruler 10 cm. below the superior border of the symphysis pubis.

2. Measurements

Diameters of inlet, midpelvis, and outlet (Fig. 238, C and D)—Normal range of anteroposterior plus transverse diameters:

Actual inlet: Anteroposterior (I-G) plus transverse (A-A′) .... 22-24 cm.

Midpelvis: Anteroposterior (M-P) plus transverse (B-B′).............. 20-22 cm.

Outlet: Anteroposterior (postsagittal, S-T) plus transverse (bituberal, C-C′) ....16-18.5 cm.

3. Source of Material

The number of patients studied is not stated by Colcher and Sussman. However, the measurements are in good agreement with those obtained in other extensive studies.

ULTRASONIC FETAL CEPHALOMETRY[†‡]

Ultrasonic fetal cephalometry is a safe and reliable method of measuring the biparietal diameter of the fetal skull in utero. Cephalopelvic relationship can be adequately assessed, using the biparietal measurement obtained by ultrasound and the interspinous diameter calculated from an anteroposterior film of the pelvis. The routine lateral film usually obtained for pelvimetry may be omitted and the radiation exposure of mother and fetus decreased thereby.

---

*This ruler, devised by Colcher and Sussman, may be obtained from the Picker X-ray Corporation, 25 South Broadway, White Plains, New York.

[†]Goldberg, B. B.; Isard, H. J.; Gershon-Cohen, J.; and Ostrum, B. J.: Radiology 87:328, 1966.

[‡]Hoffman, Von D.; Holländer, H. J.; and Weiser, P.: Gynaecologia 164:24, 1967.

RADIOLOGIC ESTIMATION OF FETAL MATURITY*

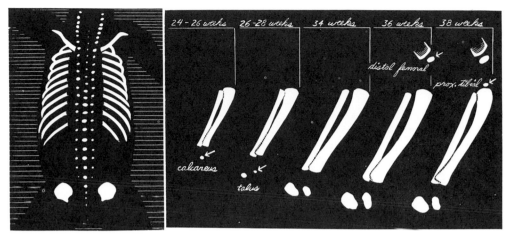

FIG. 239.–
(From Hartley, Fig. 1a.)

FIG. 240.–(From Hartley, Fig. 1b.)

1. *Technique*

   a) Central ray: Anteroposterior supine–To level of iliac crest on median plane.
   Posteroanterior prone–To level of iliac crests on median plane.
   Oblique posteroanterior–To symphysis pubis on median plane.

   b) Positions: Anteroposterior supine abdomen.
   Posteroanterior prone abdomen.
   Oblique posteroanterior abdomen.

   c) Target-film distance: Immaterial (36 inches used by Hartley).

2. *Measurements*

   Figure 239:

   10 wk. Ossification centers appear first in the transverse arches of the cervical vertebrae, subsequently appearing in the dorsal region and lumbar region. Hartley feels that the centers are never dense enough to be identified before the end of the 10th week.

   Figure 240:

   10-24 wk. Size of skull is probably the best single index of fetal age (see section on Pelvimetry, p. 274). No carpal or tarsal centers are present, and no identifiable epiphyses have yet appeared.

   24-26 wk. Calcaneous appears.

   26-28 wk. Talus appears.

   30-36 wk. Best guide is the study of developing foot ossification centers plus over-all study of skull, vertebral bodies, femora, tibiae, and soft tissues.

   36 wk. Distal femoral epiphysis appears.

   38 wk. Proximal tibial epiphysis appears.

3. *Source of Material*

   Over 10,000 cases from a large cross-section of the people in a large industrial center in Britain were studied.

*Hartley, J. B.: Brit. J. Radiol. 30:561, 1957.

FETAL WEIGHT DETERMINATION

A. Skull, Spine and Uterus Measurements to Predict Weight[*]

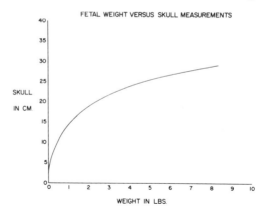

FIG. 241.—Graph showing fetal weight versus skull measurements. (From Stockland and Marks, Fig. 2.)

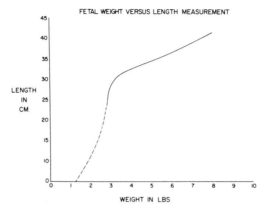

FIG. 242.—Graph showing fetal weight versus length measurements. (From Stockland and Marks, Fig. 3.)

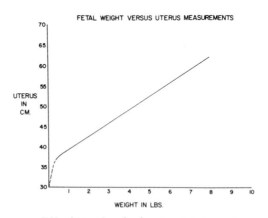

FIG. 243.—Graph showing fetal weight versus uterus measurements. (From Stockland and Marks, Fig. 4.)

[*]Stockland, L., and Marks, S. A.: Am J. Roentgenol. 86:425, 1961.

FETAL WEIGHT DETERMINATION

A. Skull, Spine and Uterus Measurements to Predict Weight

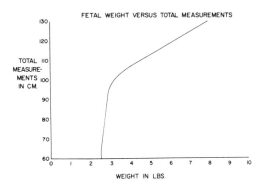

FIG. 244.—Graph showing fetal weight versus total measurements. (From Stockland and Marks, Fig. 5.)

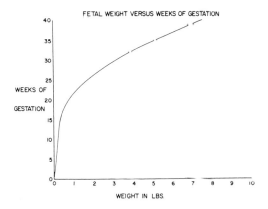

FIG. 245.—Graph showing fetal weight versus weeks of gestation. (From Stockland and Marks, Fig. 6.)

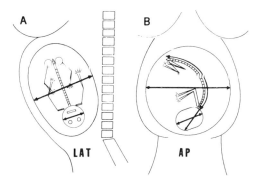

FIG. 246.—(From Stockland and Marks, Fig. 7, *A* and *B*.)

FETAL WEIGHT DETERMINATION

1. *Technique*

    a) Central ray: Anteroposterior supine — midline at level of iliac crests.

                         Lateral supine — level of iliac crest.

    b) Positions: Anteroposterior supine and lateral supine.

               Wire markers made from solder wire are taped to the abdominal wall anteriorly and along both lateral abdominal walls.

    c) Target-film distance: 40 inches.

2. *Measurements*

    a) Skull measurement. Measure biparietal diameter and occipitofrontal diameter of skull. Add the two measurements (Fig. 246, *A* and *B*). Plot total on graph (Fig. 241).

    b) Fetal length measurement. Measure length of fetal spine from coccyx to odontoid process (Fig. 246, *B*).

    c) Total length measurement. Add skull measurement and spine measurement. Plot total on graph (Fig. 242).

    d) Uterus measurement. Measure the greatest width of the uterus from the anteroposterior roentgenogram (Fig. 246, *B*) and the greatest width of the uterus from the lateral roentgenogram (Fig. 246, *A*). Add the two measurements and plot total on graph (Fig. 243).

    e) Total measurements. Add measurements of skull, total length (spine, plus skull), and uterus. Plot total on graph (Fig. 244).

    f) Average estimated weight. The weights obtained from graphs for skull, total length, uterus, and total measurement are added and averaged. This is the average, or estimated, weight on the day of roentgenography.

    g) Gestation determination. Average weight from preceding step is plotted on graph (Fig. 245) and weeks of gestation determined. From the graph the number of weeks necessary for the desired increase in the weight of the fetus can be read.

3. *Source of Material*

The results were obtained from the examinations of 50 patients and tested for accuracy on 179 patients.

B. Fetal Bone Measurements to Predict Weight*

1. *Technique*

    a) Central ray: Midline at level of iliac crest.

    b) Position: Anteroposterior supine.

    c) Target-film distance: 40 inches.

2. *Measurements*

Maximum lengths were obtained on 10 long bones: 2 femur, 2 tibia, 2 humerus, 2 radius and 2 ulna. The smaller of each pair of measurements was discarded.

Measurements were not corrected for magnification. The measurements shown below divide fetuses into two groups, with weights above or below 2,250 grams (5 lbs.). If any bone equals or exceeds the length shown the fetus is very likely to exceed 2,250 grams.

---

*Howland, W. J., and Brandfass, R. T.: Invest. Radiol. 2:61, 1967.

Bone	Measurement (cm.)
Femur	6.6
Tibia	7.0
Humerus	7.5
Ulna	6.8
Radius	5.6

(From Howland and Brandfass, Table 3.)

3. Source of Material

a) Postpartum studies were made on 60 infants within 14 days after delivery. Infant weights were between 1,500 and 3,000 grams.

b) Antepartum studies were done on 100 pelvimetry and maternal-abdomen roentgenograms obtained within 14 days before delivery. All infants weighed 1,500 to 3,000 grams at birth.

The Metric System *

The metric system had its origin in France in the year 1670. It was proposed by Gabriel Mouton, a Lyons vicar, who saw the need for a decimal system, using Latin prefixes for multiples or fractions, based upon a measurement of the earth. However, 129 years passed before official recognition was given to this system, and it was 170 years later that the metric system was adopted as the only allowable system of weights and measures in France.

In the United States, 26 more years were to pass before the Law of 1866 was passed by Congress allowing use of the metric system. In 1893 the meter and the kilogram gained recognition as the standards of length and mass by the Office of Standard Weights and Measures.

International standardization began in 1870 in Paris and led to the acceptance of the International System of Units (SI). This system has six base units, which are of defined magnitude.

Quantity	Unit	SI Symbol
Length	meter	m
Mass	kilogram	kg
Time	second	s
Electric current	ampere	A
Thermodynamic temperature	degree Kelvin	°K
Luminous intensity	candela	cd

All other quantities are derived from these six using, when desired, the following prefixes or multipliers:

Multiplication Factor[†]		Prefix[‡]	SI Symbol
1 000 000	$= 10^6$	mega	M
1 000	$= 10^3$	kilo	k
100	$= 10^2$	hecto	h
10	$= 10^1$	deka	da
0.1	$= 10^{-1}$	deci	d
0.01	$= 10^{-2}$	centi	c
0.001	$= 10^{-3}$	milli	m
0.000 001	$= 10^{-6}$	micro	μ
0.000 000 001	$= 10^{-9}$	nano	n
0.000 000 000 001	$= 10^{-12}$	pico	p

[†]Abbreviated list.

[‡]When these prefixes are used to form new unit designations only one prefix is used at a time.

Thus instead of millimicrogram (mμg), nanogram (ng) would be used and micromicron ($\mu\mu$) would become picometer (pm). Unit designations should consist of a single prefix

*Reprinted from The Journal of Bone and Joint Surgery with permission of the editor and the publisher. The material was prepared by Albert H. Burstein, Ph.D.

to designate a multiplier and a single suffix to describe the physical quantity to which the multiplier is applied. Thus micrometers (μm) is preferred to microns (μ).

The unit of *force* in the SI system is the *newton* (N) which is the force required to give *one* kilogram of mass an acceleration of *one* meter per second per second. However, in engineering and the physical sciences in this country the accepted practice is to use the kilogram-force (kgf) which is defined as the force required to accelerate *one* kilogram of mass (kg) 9.80665 meters per second per second. A kilogram-force is approximately equal to the weight of a kilogram of mass. (The gravitational acceleration varies 0.5 per cent over the surface of the earth.)

A modified system which differs from the SI system in that it uses kilogram-force instead of newtons may be useful as a transition system. It is suggested that if this modified system is used, a footnote of the following form appear in the publications in which the unit "kilogram-force" (kgf) appears:

A kilogram-force (kgf) is exactly equal to 9.80665 newtons (N) and approximately equal to the weight of a kilogram (kg) of mass.

The use of the newton as the unit of force is certainly preferable, but the use of the kgf can be accepted to allow an easier transition to the SI system.

The old c.g.s. system, since it is one of the most familiar metric systems, is compared with the SI system and the modified metric system just described in the following table. Subsequent tables give the conversion factors for the commonly used units of measure.

COMPARISON OF BASIC UNITS

	c.g.s.	SI[1]	Modified Metric[2]
Mass	gram (gm)	kilogram (kg)	kilogram (kg)
Length	centimeter (cm)	meter (m)	meter (m)
Time	second (s)	second (s)	second (s)
Force	dyne[3]	newton (N)[4]	kilogram-force (kgf)[5]

[1]Le Systeme International d'Unites, which is called the SI system, is used by most countries of the world as the official system of weights and measures and is the preferred system.

[2]The Modified Metric system is acceptable as an interim or transitional system.

[3]A dyne is the force required to give a free mass of one gram an acceleration of one centimeter per second per second.

[4]A newton is the force required to give a free mass of one kilogram an acceleration of one meter per second per second.

[5]A kilogram-force is the force required to give a free mass of one kilogram an acceleration of 9.80665* meters per second per second. This acceleration is the International standard gravity value ("standard acceleration"). Therefore, 1 *kilogram-force* (kgf) is *approximately* equivalent to the *weight* of a 1 *kilogram* (kg) *mass*, since the value of gravity varies 0.5% over the earth's surface.

$$(1 \text{ kilogram-force} = 9.80665 \text{ newtons*}$$
$$1 \text{ kilogram-force} = 9.80665 \times 10^5 \text{ dynes*})$$

(The term kilopond has been used to mean kilogram-force.)
A gram-force (gmf) is defined by: 1000 gmf = 1 kgf.

---

*Exact conversion; that is, all subsequent digits are zeros.

CONVERSION FACTORS

LENGTH

Equivalences:

angstrom = 1×10^{-10} meter (0. 0 000 000 001 m)
millimicron* = 1×10^{-9} meter (0.000 000 001 m)
micron (micrometer) = 1×10^{-6} meter (0.000 001 m)

To convert from	To	Multiply by
inches	meters	0.0254[†]
feet	meters	0.30480[†]
yards	meters	0.91440[†]
miles	kilometers	1.6093

AREA

To convert from	To	Multiply by
square inches	square meters	0.000 64516[†]
square feet	square meters	.092903

VOLUME

Definition:

1 liter = 0.001[†] cubic meter or one cubic decimeter (dm^3)
(1 milliliter = 1[†] cubic centimeter)

To convert from	To	Multiply by
cubic inches	cubic centimeters	16.387
ounces (U.S. fluid)	cubic centimeters	29.574
ounces (Brit. fluid)	cubic centimeters	28.413
pints (U.S. fluid)	cubic centimeters	473.18
pints (Brit. fluid)	cubic centimeters	568.26
cubic feet	cubic meters	0.028317

MASS

To convert from	To	Multiply by
pounds (avdp.)	kilograms	0.45359
slugs[‡]	kilograms	14.594

FORCE

To convert from	To	Multiply by
ounces-force (ozf)	newtons	0.27802
ounces-force (ozf)	kilogram-force	0.028350
pounds-force (lbf)	newtons	4.4732
pounds-force (lbf)	kilogram-force	0.45359

---

*This double-prefix usage is not desirable. This unit is actually a nanometer (10^{-9} meter = 10^{-7} centimeter).

[†]Exact conversion; that is, all subsequent digits are zeros.

[‡]A slug is a unit of mass which if acted on by a force of one pound will have an acceleration of one foot per second per second.

STRESS (OR PRESSURE)

To convert from	To	Multiply by
pounds-force/square inch (psi)	newton/square meter	6894.8
pounds-force/square inch (psi)	newton/square centimeter	0.68948
pounds-force/square inch (psi)	kilogram-force/square centimeter	0.070307

TORQUE (OR MOMENT)

To convert from	To	Multiply by
pound-force·feet	newton meter	1.3559
pound-force·feet	kilogram-force·meters	0.13826

ENERGY (OR WORK)

Definition:

1 joule (J) is the work done by a one-newton force moving through a displacement of one meter in the direction of the force.

1 cal (gm) = 4.1840 joules

To convert from	To	Multiply by
foot·pounds-force	joules	1.3559
foot·pounds-force	meter·kilogram-force	0.13826
ergs	joules	1×10^{-7} [†]
b.t.u.	cal (gm)	252.00
foot·pounds-force	cal (gm)	0.32405

TEMPERATURE CONVERSION TABLE

$$°C = \frac{°F - 32}{1.8}$$

°F	°C
98.6	37
99	37.2
99.5	37.5
100	37.8
100.5	38.1
101	38.3
101.5	38.6
102	38.9
102.5	39.2
103	39.4
103.5	39.7
104	40.0

References

U.S. Department of Commerce, National Bureau of Standards: *Units of Weights and Measures*, Pub. 286, May 1967; *National Bureau of Standards Handbook 102, ASTM Metric Practice Guide*, 2nd ed., March 1967.

Ritchie-Calder, P. R.: Scient. Am. 223:17, 1970. (Overview of the problem of metric conversion.)

Index

INDEX